Riddles in Accountable Healthcare

A Primer to develop analytic intuition for medical homes and population health

Eran Bellin

Copyright © 2015 Eran Bellin
All rights reserved.

ISBN: 1503053873
ISBN 13: 9781503053878
Library of Congress Control Number: 2014919449
CreateSpace Independent Publishing Platform
North Charleston, South Carolina

Dedication

To the associates of Montefiore Medical Center, who are daily transforming our organization into an ever-better steward of population health.

To my father, Lowell Bellin, who introduced me to public health and communal responsibility.

To my mother, Talah Bellin, who encouraged careful thought and clear exposition.

Contents

Preface · xi
Introduction · xiii

Solving Riddles in Healthcare

Chapter 1 How I Solve Accountable Healthcare Riddles
Clinical Looking Glass—Temporally Aware
Cohort Builder · 3

Chapter 2 How Great is Our Reputation?
The Wrong Question Answered Carefully Can Clarify
Our Values · 7

**Chapter 3 How Do You Know if Your Healthcare System is
Right-Sized?** · 11

Preventing Readmissions

**Chapter 4 Does Visiting Your Doctor after Hospital Discharge
Prevent Hospital Readmission?**
Or Is Seeing Your Doctor Dangerous? · · · · · · · · · · · · · · · 23

Chapter 5 Heads or Tails—Which End is Up?
Choosing Between Two Sides of a Durational Event · · · · · 29

Chapter 6 Does My Regional Health Information Organization Prevent Hospital Admissions? · 33

Chapter 7 How Could Your Privacy Decisions Impact My RHIO Experience?
Don't Silence My Silence · 37

ACCOUNTABILITY

Chapter 8 Am I My Brother's Keeper?
The New Longitudinal Healthcare Paradigm · · · · · · · · · 41

Chapter 9 To Corrupt Man
An Impossible Goal, Inadequate Surveillance, Harsh Punishment, and a Failure of Integrity and Leadership Promote the Dishonorable · 45

Chapter 10 I Am Not Responsible Until I Say I Am
The Folly of Reliance on Unexamined Billing Processes · 51

Chapter 11 Who Is Responsible for the Events of the Hospitalization? · 55

DATA ANALYTICS AND PREDICTIVE MODELS

Chapter 12 Epidemic of Diastolic Dysfunction in the Bronx
Knowing the Source Is Half the Battle · · · · · · · · · · · · · · 59

Chapter 13 Predictive Analytic Surprise
How Good Care Confounds Biologic Intuition in Building Predictive Models · 63

Chapter 14 Can We Learn from One Another?
Do We Have to Validate Each Study in Our Own Environment? · 67

Chapter 15 Adjustment or Excuse?
  What Happens When You Adjust for Race? · · · · · · · · · · 71

Chapter 16 Why Am I Doing Better than You in Each of My Subgroups, but Overall You Are Looking Better than Me?
  Simpson's Paradox · 73

Developing Longitudinal Intuition

Chapter 17 Does Zero Mean Never?
  How the Question, Its Context, and Statistics Drive Judgment · 79

Chapter 18 Will I Be Able to Play the Piano?
  Worse Disease Gets Better Outcome
  Cull the Herd and Leave Only the Strong · · · · · · · · · · · 87

Chapter 19 Paradoxical Worsening of Metrics as Care Innovation and Implementation Improves Quality
  A Cautionary Tale in Deep Venous Thrombosis · · · · · · · 91

Chapter 20 But It Makes Biologic Sense…
  The Illusion of the Known: "It isn't what we don't know that gives us trouble. It's what we know that ain't so."
  —Will Rogers · 93

Chapter 21 An Epidemic of Hypercalcemia
  "Once you eliminate the impossible, whatever remains, no matter how improbable, must be the truth."
  —Sherlock Holmes · 97

Chapter 22 Big Is Better? But Is It Enough? · · · · · · · · · · · · · · · · · · · 101

Population Health
The Socioeconomic Status Trilogy

Chapter 23 Does Low Socioeconomic Status Predispose to Higher Readmission Rate?
How Intervention Thwarts Attribution with No Good Deed Going Unpunished ·················· 109
    Appendix 1: Group Definition in Cohort-Builder Clinical Looking Glass ····················· 118
    Appendix 2: Single-Created Variable to Represent Socioeconomic Status ····················· 119

Chapter 24 I Am Too Poor to Benefit from SES Improvement
Threshold in the Service of Understanding ········· 121

Chapter 25 Inadequate Power Obscures Findings ··············· 125

The Obesity Epidemic Trilogy

Chapter 26 Where All the Children Are Above Average
Lake Wobegon Meets Public Health ·············· 133

Chapter 27 Belching Fat
Fat Pollution—the Modern Scourge of High BMI ····· 137

Chapter 28 How Can We Be Getting Fatter When a Higher Percentage is Losing Weight? ····················· 141

Silencing Death – The Unsolved Riddle

Chapter 29 When the Dead Are Silenced, Who Speaks for the Living?
Blind to One Million US Dead—How Public Policy for Healthcare Is Thwarted ······················ 145

ABOUT
About Advanced Analytics · 153
About Me · 155

EPILOGUE: ABOUT MONTEFIORE MEDICAL CENTER, BRONX, NEW YORK · 159
BIBLIOGRAPHY · 161

Preface

IN THE UNITED STATES, accountable healthcare, with measurable improved health outcomes, is the purpose of all healthcare expenditures. If we are to follow a group of patients to an agreed-upon outcome, we must work to develop our analytic skills and intuition. Such wisdom is earned through years of making mistakes, together with a willingness to learn from them.

Riddles in Accountable Healthcare is a quick-start guide for those wishing to develop longitudinal healthcare analytic intuition. Using real-world examples with data occasionally modified to make the instructive point, this book explores questions raised by analysts who have worked in a medical center committed to longitudinal population health. I am inspired by the writers Berton Rouché,[1] Stephen Dubner,[2] and Malcolm Gladwell,[3,4] who have shown that important truths can be transmitted through engaging and insightful vignettes.

I hope that this book will find a receptive audience not only in schools and with practitioners of public health, health administration, medicine, and nursing, but also with members of the general public who are interested in understanding issues that drive policy decisions in healthcare—an industry that consumes 18 percent of the US gross national product.

Eran Bellin, MD

January 20, 2015

Introduction

IN 2007 THE US government instituted the Physician Quality Reporting Initiative as a voluntary program to encourage physicians to provide better care by following specific medical guidelines. By first providing a "carrot" of increased dollars, the initiative was designed to encourage doctors to change their practices before the eventual "stick" in later years of financial penalties for not following the guidelines. Thus, through a combination of legislation and financial incentives, the federal government had essentially decided it would practice medicine.

Notable among the guidelines was a protocol for the management of pneumonia in emergency rooms. This measure required every pneumonia patient be treated with antibiotics immediately in the ER before even reaching the hospital floor. To the average onlooker, this seemed like a good idea. If you were sick enough to be hospitalized, the conventional wisdom said, you should get your medicine as soon as possible. You should not have to wait for hours in the ER and then for hours in a hospital bed before receiving lifesaving antibiotics.

The National Committee for Quality Assurance (NCQA), the American College of Emergency Physicians, and the American Medical Association's consortium for Performance Improvement all endorsed the pneumonia treatment guideline, also known as Physician Quality Reporting System Measure (PQRS) #59. By 2009, 11 percent of eligible providers were reporting on their compliance.

Yet in January 2013, PQRS #59 was retired. Why?

Its retirement was not an indication of its success. Retirement, in this case, was an indication that the guideline had gone wrong—terribly wrong. Critics of the measure accused it of distorting medical judgment, encouraging irresponsible prescribing practices, and potentially contributing to the emergence of superbugs—infections highly resistant to antibiotics.

What error led the medical community to this unfortunate guideline?

A published study had shown that early antibiotic therapy saved lives.[5] However, the guideline writers approached the article without a full awareness of time—without what I think of as temporal intelligence. The study identified pneumonia patients from discharge diagnoses and reported that those patients who had been treated with antibiotics in the ER had a lower death rate. The guideline writers surmised that by requiring antibiotic administration for pneumonia patients in the ER, doctors could achieve better results in a larger population.

Regrettably, they failed to recognize that emergency physicians experience "time's arrow" in the forward direction. ER physicians confront diagnostic uncertainty in the narrow window of time available to them to evaluate a patient.[6] Only 50 percent of those affirmatively diagnosed with pneumonia are known to have it in the emergency room. Discharge diagnoses are determined at the date of discharge and entered into the medical record by billing clerks four to seven days after discharge. Therefore, the only way ER physicians could possibly achieve the 100 percent compliance required by the guideline was to treat everyone in the ER with an antibiotic—a requirement impossible to achieve without wasteful and potentially dangerous exposure of large numbers of patients to unneeded antibiotics.

The organization of medical care is changing in the United States with more accountability for the long-term outcome. For those who build policy as well as for those who implement programs, an understanding of how to think about new questions is critical to planning, implementation, evaluation, and learning from errors.

This book is designed to expose the reader to "riddles"—questions whose answers become crucial as we try to determine what we should measure and what we should learn from what we measure. *Riddles* is written in a discursive, engaging style to encourage you to develop deep intuition, whether you make healthcare policy, are subject to it, or pay for it. It should therefore be of value to everyone.

Solving Riddles in Healthcare

1

How I Solve Accountable Healthcare Riddles

Clinical Looking Glass—Temporally Aware Cohort Builder

TO BE ACCOUNTABLE AS a medical professional, you first have to decide: "Accountable for whom"? You have to identify the relevant patients by their intrinsic characteristics measurable at one point in time (age, gender, race), and by their experiences or findings related in time. Relating findings temporally establishes a case definition. For example, a case definition for elevated blood pressure might be established by finding an elevated blood pressure in an outpatient visit in 2013 with another elevated blood pressure within a year of the first. The second elevated blood pressure marks the patient with the hypertension diagnosis from that moment on.

"That moment on" is an important concept. That moment is the "index date: time" from which all subsequent analyses will begin for that patient. How rapidly did your chronic hypertensive patients come under control? How many of your chronic hypertensives were hospitalized in the year subsequent to the time they were established as chronic hypertensives? These are simple questions, and you might ask why not just use a billing code to establish the start time. You are free to do that, but questions using rich clinical data of the electronic medical record can be much more clinically refined.

Consider the following two scenarios, which highlight the possible refinement:

Scenario #1:

Find all patients admitted to the hospital in 2014 with (1) diagnoses of congestive heart failure, (2) who in the six months prior to admission had a cardiac echo with an ejection fraction of less than thirty-five, and (3) within thirty days of discharge from the hospital were started on enalapril. The final step would be to follow these patients from the moment of prescription to first hospitalization in the subsequent year. Do the same for another drug and compare the results.

Scenario #2:

Find all patients who had diagnoses of atrial fibrillation for the first time in 2013, either in a hospital, during an outpatient visit, or during an emergency department visit. Make sure that there were no other diagnoses of atrial fibrillation in the previous ten years. The patients who fit this description become the incident atrial fibrillation group in 2013. Identify three subgroups and study them for two years. One subgroup is never prescribed oral anticoagulants outside of the hospital. A second subgroup is prescribed dabigatrin but never warfarin. A third subgroup is prescribed warfarin but not any other oral anticoagulant over the next two years.

Now follow each of these three groups to an outcome—the members' deaths.

What is the index date for each of the three subgroups from which you look for elapsed time until death?

For those who started on a specific anticoagulant, the index date: time would be the date of the first prescription. For those not started on any anticoagulant, the index date: time would be the date: time of first atrial fibrillation diagnosis.

Notice the richness of possibilities in your questions and analyses.

You need a temporally aware cohort builder to create the relevant patient groups, identify their index dates, and relate those cohorts to interesting target outcomes. These target outcomes themselves may be qualified by intricate temporal relationships.

Just collecting data in a data warehouse or having software that filters or slices and dices data does not create these opportunities for temporal analysis.[7] When Montefiore Medical Center could not find a commercial system to suit our needs, we built our own.

For fifteen years, spending more than $40 million, and with twenty-two staff directly employed, Clinical Looking Glass[8] (CLG) was built at the Montefiore Medical Center. Our cohort builder sits on top of the electronic medical record data, collecting both inpatient and outpatient data. Data goes back to April 1997 and contains information on more than 2.4 million unique patients. To better understand the breadth of patient population found in CLG, I developed a concept that I call "touched by Montefiore's information system." Patients are considered "touched by Montefiore" if they have laboratory tests, medication prescriptions, emergency department or outpatient visits, or hospital admissions. In 2013, in the borough of the Bronx, New York, with 1.4 million residents, 492,993 unique patients were touched.

A separate instance of CLG supports the Bronx Regional Health Information organization, which provides Bronx-wide healthcare analytics.

Because CLG can perform temporal analyses internally without needing to postprocess for external temporal analyses[7], it supports analyses in the deidentified mode (protecting patient privacy). For those with a need-to-know and privilege, it can reveal patient names for healthcare interventions, making it a perfect tool for proactive healthcare management. When patient identity is requested, the system records the name of the requester, the date, and the question being asked for future audits.

At Montefiore, CLG training has been integrated for more than seven years with the internal medicine residency program affording first-year residents the opportunity to gain an understanding of longitudinal healthcare responsibility and the potential for quality improvement projects and research. Training in CLG is widespread among pathology residents and cardiology fellows who participate in CLG boot camps, and Clinical Research Training Program fellows at the Albert Einstein College of Medicine. More than eight hundred people have been trained to date.

In October 2013 Montefiore Medical Center sold commercialization rights for CLG to Streamline Health (in Atlanta, Georgia), which markets it under the name Looking Glass. We look forward to working with colleagues in other institutions to compare longitudinal analyses in the near future.

2

How Great is Our Reputation?

The Wrong Question Answered Carefully Can Clarify Our Values

CONCERN FOR OUR OWN reputation is a common human trait. Observe how often we see best-of lists in the media for restaurants, colleges—and hospitals. Yes, it is only human nature to want to be the best, but in healthcare it is not always clear how such a metric is created. For instance, is "best hospital" based on low mortality rate? Or is the concept of best built upon tasty hospital food and excellent parking? Is best determined by the reputation of the institution?

One way to assess a hospital's reputation is to ask other physicians what they really think of the institution. This is a classic popularity contest where people in the know are tasked with assigning a reputational value for each hospital on a scale of one to ten, averaging the scores for each hospital and sorting the institutions accordingly. You might be surprised to realize how many of the best-of lists use some variant of this high school popularity contest methodology to establish reputational primacy!

A more objective measure might be to look at all the patients who are admitted to a hospital for specific procedures or care and evaluate how far those patients travel to obtain services from that institution. The distribution of distances can give a sense of how much effort these patients are willing to expend to obtain care. The farther they travel, the more compelling that hospital's reputation must be. Do princes of Saudi Arabia fly to this facility to get their care? They fly to the Mayo Clinic.

For example, to evaluate the cardiology reputation of your hospital, you might take all the cardiology patients who underwent cardiac catheterization at your hospital, look at their addresses, map the distance from their homes to your institution with a mapping program like Google Maps, and then organize the patients in order of distance from the hospital. You can then display characteristic percentiles of distance, and can compare the change over time in the distance values in each percentile. This will determine reputational change (see table 1 for an example).

Table 1. Reputational change using distance percentiles, Montefiore Medical Center

	10th Percentile	25th Percentile	50th Percentile	75th Percentile	90th Percentile
Year					
2005	1.86 miles	3.02 miles	5.02 miles	8.11 miles	66.82 miles
2013	1.69 miles	2.85 miles	4.73 miles	6.88 miles	13.09 miles

In 2005 the 25th percentile had a distance of 3.02 miles. This means that 25 percent of patients had a home-to-hospital distance of 3.02 miles or less. The 75th percentile was 8.11 miles. This means that 75 percent of the 2005 patients with cardiac procedures had their home located 8.11 miles or less from the hospital.

Now observe that for each percentile in 2013, the distance was smaller than in 2005. In 2013, the 75th percentile distance was 6.88 miles versus 8.11 miles in 2005. This means that people who had these procedures lived closer to the hospital in 2013 than in 2005. We are not drawing from a larger geographic area. We have not increased our geographic reputational footprint.

Is there another reputational metric? Perhaps if patients with greater wealth select our hospital, then it can be surmised that those with financial wherewithal—and the power to choose—are affirming our good reputation. As Tevye, the milkman, sang in *Fiddler on the Roof*, "When you're rich, they think you really know."[9] It is possible to take advantage of census data to build a neighborhood metric of socioeconomic status (SES)[10] and assign to each address the SES of its neighborhood. Since our hospital is in New York State, we will scale the values so that if a patient's neighborhood were assigned a score of zero, his or her SES would be at New York State's average. The units of measure will be in standard deviations—a measure of variability whose detail I will spare you. However, a negative multiple of standard deviation units is equivalent to saying that the neighborhood is poorer than New York State's average. A positive multiple of standard deviation units is equivalent to saying the neighborhood is wealthier than the New York State average.

Using the neighborhood SES metric for Montefiore Medical Center, it is possible to observe the following about the cardiology patients who underwent cardiac catheterization (see table 2).

Table 2. Socioeconomic index, Montefiore Medical Center

	10th Percentile	25th Percentile	50th Percentile	75th Percentile	90th Percentile
Year					
2005	-6.89	-4.07	-1.37	-0.264	1.07
2013	-7.09	-5.06	-2.01	-0.597	0.712

Note: These are units of standard deviation of the New York State mean.

First, the big picture: Montefiore Medical Center's population is quite poor compared to others in New York State. Even at the 75th percentile, our patients are poorer than the New York State average (SES < 0). In other words, 75 percent of our patients are poorer than the New York State average.

You can also see that in 2005, each percentile was wealthier than in 2013. Our hospital does not seem to be attracting a richer clientele.

So now for the critical question: Have we failed? Are we poorer in reputation? Should we shamefacedly close up shop?

One possible response is that this metric is the correct metric, but real reputational improvement should be sought in the extreme, most complex cases drawn from the top 5 percent of the population, not the lower ranges. It would be necessary to look at the 95th percentile for distance to draw an inference of whether our reputation is improving.

Along the same lines of reasoning, it is possible that too many prosaic procedures were included, and not the cutting-edge ones where our reputational enhancement would shine.

Ultimately, however, distance popularity as a metric of central worth must be rejected because it asks the wrong question. The Montefiore data is telling us that we care for people who live close to us—not too shabby. We care for the Bronx community, many of whom live far below the New York State average SES. Montefiore's chief executive officer, as a matter of pride, used to say that from the hospital rooftop we could see the families we serve. Our demonstration of excellence is based upon the quality of service we deliver to our Bronx family, not the number of people from foreign lands we can attract.

> "For what shall it profit a man, if he shall gain the whole world, and lose his own soul?"—Mark 8:36.

3

How Do You Know if Your Healthcare System is Right-Sized?

Emergency Department "Dwell Time" as Evidence of Right-Sizing Healthcare Delivery Systems

AS UNITED STATES SOCIETY centralizes responsibility for healthcare access and delivery through increased subsidized entitlements, assessing sufficient resources becomes of central concern. The invisible hand of the free market no longer drives the distribution of this communal benefit. With healthcare transformed into a publicly acknowledged right, measurement of healthcare access becomes a matter of public policy, concern, and equity.

Question: Do Americans have enough healthcare resources in their communities to satisfy their needs?

Answer: Medical need is a complex notion—merging the emergent, urgent, reparative, preventive, and cosmetic. Patient desires, satisfaction, sense of entitlement, and resource access all drive utilization.

So, is there a meaningful single summary metric?

Seeking a single, all-encompassing metric is naive in the extreme. Consider the preventive medicine domain. Tracking colonoscopy screening for colon cancer, mammography for breast cancer, and hypertension control for stroke and heart-attack prevention require multiple metrics.

Recognizing the impossibility of a single metric, this chapter focuses on satisfaction of perceived need. Patients presenting at an emergency room subject themselves to multiple inconveniences, so their very presence is a public declaration of perceived need for urgent or emergent care. In some communities, the ER becomes a site of primary care, with encounters that could have been prevented had there been adequate, affordable, and accessible primary care.

How does the study of emergency room dynamics provide insight?

Emergency room doctors should be diagnosing, stabilizing, and admitting patients who need admission to the hospital. If there are not enough beds in the hospital attached to the emergency room, then ER traffic backs up. Unable to discharge patients into the hospital, ER doctors' primary functions are degraded as they take on the ongoing management of patients who should have been admitted. As a result, the efficiency of the primary ER process also deteriorates.

If there is not enough access to primary care doctors in a community, the emergency department picks up the slack. If there are no strategies in place to move patients who are unsafe at home to an available nursing home or a neighboring hospital, the ER becomes a holding facility with resultant efficiency degradation.

Dwell time in the ER—the time between triage and discharge, whether to a hospital bed or to home—is a potential metric for adequacy of a healthcare delivery system that accommodates patients' perceived needs.

Patients who are ultimately admitted to a hospital first spend time in the ER for evaluation and acute management, and then they wait for an available bed. Some of the dwell time is inherent in the processes of the emergency room itself—diagnosis and stabilization. But when an increased number of people overwhelm an emergency room—due to any of the causes described above—the dwell time prior to admission lengthens. Consider two hypothetical populations of ER patients who are ultimately admitted to the hospital: one group in 2005 and one in 2013 (see figure 1).

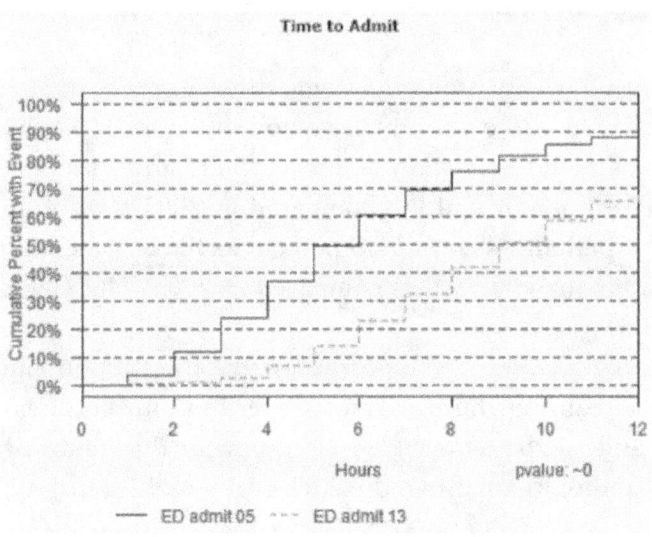

Year	1 hour	2 hours	4 hours	8 hours	12 hours
2005	3.8% (3.5, 4.0)*	11.9% (11.5, 12.3)	36.9% (36.4, 37.5)	75.9% (75.4, 76.4)	89.1% (88.7, 89.4)
2013	0.3% (0.3, 0.4)	0.9% (0.8, 1.0)	7.1% (6.8, 7.3)	42.0% (41.5, 42.5)	68.2% (67.7, 68.7)

Note: Parentheses include a range of values built by a statistical model.

Figure 1. Cumulative percentage admitted by hours measured from ER triage to hospital admission.

On the *x*-axis is the number of hours that elapsed from triage until admission. The *y*-axis has the cumulative percentage of patients admitted by that elapsed time.

In 2005, by four hours after ER triage, 36.9 percent of patients had been admitted. By eight hours, 75.9 percent had been admitted. In 2013, 7.1 percent had been admitted by four hours, and 42 percent had been admitted by eight hours. As you can see, a smaller proportion of patients were admitted in 2013 by four and eight hours than in 2005. Dwell time increased from 2005 to 2013, with a highly significant p value (*pvalue* ~0), suggesting a deterioration of the dwell time metric over this time period.

If our metric focused on a single time cut point such as cumulative percentage admitted within twelve hours (an overly forgiving goal that none of us would personally endorse), the relative risk of admission before twelve hours in 2013 as compared to 2005 is 0.766 (0.752, 0.779). In 2013 a patient was only 76.6 percent as likely to be admitted before twelve hours had elapsed as compared to 2005. This suggests a significant deterioration.

You might consider the possibility that the ER population changed over time, causing the dwell time deterioration, but a careful look at gender and age breakdowns reveal no major difference over time (see tables 3 and 4). If anything, the 2013 group looks younger.

Table 3. ER patients admitted by gender and year at Montefiore Medical Center

	Male	Female
2005	12,539 (43%)	16,884 (57%)
2013	14,868 (44%)	18,960 (56%)

Table 4. Age Percentiles of emergency department patients admitted by year

	10th Percentile	25th Percentile	50th Percentile	75th Percentile	90th Percentile
Year					
2005	10	35	56	73	84
2013	9	33	56	71	83

Another group serviced in the ER are those who are ultimately determined not to require admission and thus are sent home. In figure 2 is the dwell time analysis for patients who ultimately were not admitted to the hospital.

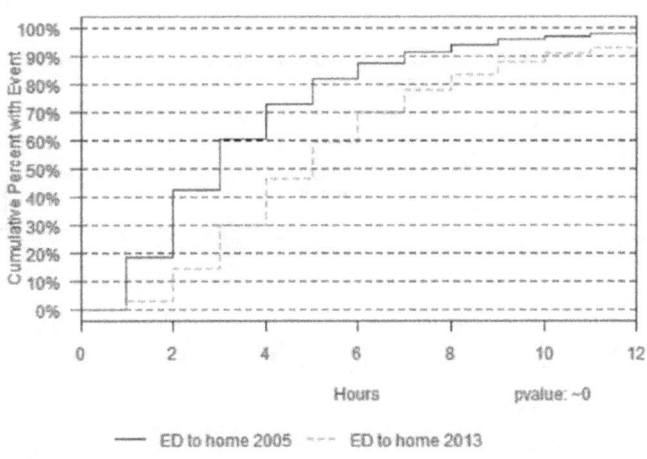

	By 1 hour	By 2 hours	By 4 hours	By 8 hours	By 12 hours
2005	18.6% (18.3, 18.8)	42.4% (42.1, 42.7)	73.1% (72.8, 73.4)	94.0% (93.9, 94.2)	97.9% (97.8, 98.0)
2013	3.1% (3.0, 3.2)	14.4% (14.2, 14.6)	46.2% (45.9, 46.5)	83.6% (83.4, 83.9)	93.7% (93.5, 93.8)

Figure 2. Cumulative percentage of patients discharged, by hours from ER triage to discharge

By four hours, 73.1 percent of the patients had been discharged to home in 2005, while in 2013 only 46.2 percent had been discharged. Once again, there is a significant deterioration of the dwell time metric. For people who were not admitted, the overall inefficiencies engendered in admission traffic back up affected them as well.

As seen in tables 5 and 6, the demographics for those discharged to home reveal similar proportions of men and women, and an older population in 2013 than 2005.

Table 5. Number and percentage of discharged ER patients by gender

	Male	Female
2005	44,517 (43%)	58,973 (57%)
2013	50,473 (43%)	67,547 (57%)

Table 6. Age Percentiles of ER patients discharged to home, by year

	10th Percentile	25th Percentile	50th Percentile	75th Percentile	90th Percentile
Year					
2005	1.9	7	24	44	60
2013	2.5	9	27	48	62

Of course, one might explain the dwell time deterioration by restating the claim of changing population characteristics. The patient population has gotten sicker in ways not captured by simple gender or age distribution. This argument claims that the worsening dwell time is not due to internal process failures but to factors intrinsic to the recent patient population.

Question: How would you reject this self-serving argument?

Answer: You could establish a control emergency department. This emergency department would ideally be in the same geographic area and have patients with the same range of clinical problems, but not be attached to a single hospital. This freestanding emergency unit would transfer its admission-eligible patients to a number of hospitals in the geographic area. Its dwell time would be reflective of the time it takes to do the primary work of the emergency room itself, as the backup of patients in any single hospital would not be rate limiting to its ER discharges for hospital admission.

Such a freestanding emergency room was set up within five miles of Montefiore, but it was designed to use capacity at multiple hospitals to facilitate admissions for those Montefiore doctors deemed in need of hospital admissions.

Figure 3 compare the time to admission metric between the freestanding emergency department (ED) and the adjacent emergency department from January to March 2014.

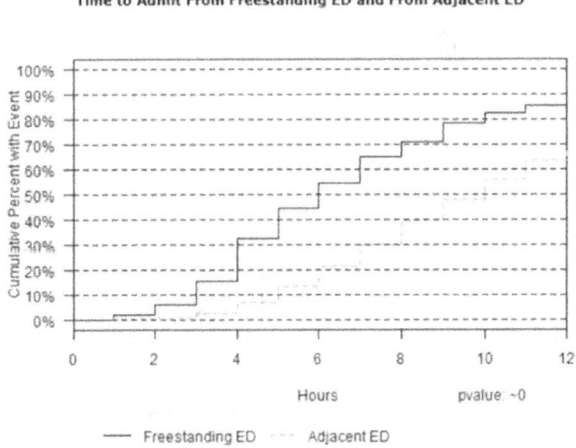

	By 1 hour	By 2 hours	By 4 hours	By 8 hours	By 12 hours
Freestanding ED	2.1%	6.2%	32.3%	70.9%	86.6%
	(0.5, 3.6)	(3.6, 8.8)	(27.2, 37.2)	(65.6, 75.4)	(82.5, 89.8)
Adjacent ED	0.3%	0.9%	6.9%	39.2%	66.7%
	(0.2, 0.5)	(0.7, 1.1)	(6.3, 7.4)	(38.2, 40.3)	(65.7, 67.7)

Figure 3. Freestanding versus adjacent ED, cumulative percentage admitted to hospital in hours from triage to admission

As can be seen, the freestanding ED stabilized and discharged patients to an admission site dramatically faster than the ED adjacent to the hospital. At four hours, the adjacent ED had admitted only 6.9 percent of its patients, while the freestanding ED had admitted 32.3 percent.

We found in the adjacent ED, a higher proportion of males and similar aged patients (Tables 7,8).

Table 7. Gender of patients discharged to a hospital by freestanding versus adjacent ED

	Male	Female
Freestanding ED	138 (41%)	199 (59%)
Adjacent ED	3,668 (44%)	4,615 (56%)

Table 8. Age percentiles by freestanding versus adjacent ED

	10th Percentile	25th Percentile	50th Percentile	75th Percentile	90th Percentile
ED Type					
Freestanding	23	34	53	72	83
Adjacent	8	33	56	71	82

Further analysis revealed that the freestanding ED bested the hospital-adjacent ED by discharging two-thirds (206 of 308) of its patients into an underpopulated hospital not originally part of the Montefiore hospital system.

In truth, I did not calculate time until the patient actually arrived on the hospital floor of the nonadjacent hospital, but the point is intriguing. The proper shifting of our admissions to available hospital beds, even when they are not necessarily the beds nearest to our ED, is a desirable strategy, assuming we have the concurrence of both the families and their clinicians. Additional strategies will be found when federal financing meets administrative creativity, such as directing patients who cannot be left at home alone to nursing homes for short periods of nonhospital supervised care.

Building urgent care center capacity, primary care capacity, and timely primary follow-up care may reduce emergency room visits, overcrowding, and concomitant efficiency degradation. It is important, however, to be cautious in assuming that improving service at the emergency room portal, will reduce dwell time.

The example of New York City toll roads and bridges may be instructive in this caution.

In *The Power Broker*, Robert Caro[11] reported that as New York City improved its roads, widened its highways, and built bridges to reduce traffic congestion in the 1920s and 1930s, people were encouraged to move out to the suburbs. The increasing suburban population generated more traffic heading into the city for work and fun, eventually re-creating the traffic jams these public works were built to address.

In this same vein, some ER services may create rather than satisfy demand. To what extent this may happen is unclear. One hopes that illness is not in inexhaustible supply, and that it is possible to meet true demand with proper regional bed management, primary care, and urgent care center availability.

Preventing Readmissions

4

Does Visiting Your Doctor after Hospital Discharge Prevent Hospital Readmission?

Or is Seeing Your Doctor Dangerous?

WHEN YOU ARE VERY sick, it stands to reason that you need to go to the hospital. You hope that your medical complaint will be resolved by the time you are discharged. You also expect that, for any outstanding issue, your clinician will have developed a plan coordinating your care after hospital discharge to prevent an unnecessary readmission.

A fraction of the hospital readmissions that occur within thirty days of hospital discharge are thought to be preventable. Jencks et al.[12] reviewed Medicare fee-for-service claims, noting in 2009 that more than half of Medicare patients who were readmitted within thirty days of hospital discharge did not have a visit with their physician in the interim.

These authors claimed that this perceived lapse suggested a considerable opportunity for improvement.

Question: Is this a correct reading of the situation?

Answer: On the surface, Jencks et al.'s conclusion seems reasonable. It fits together nicely with the notion that a visit with a doctor could mitigate problems, particularly in complicated cases. If these problems are remediated, so the argument goes, an unnecessary hospital readmission could be prevented. Of course, this hypothesis assumes that the doctor will seek, find, and offer an effective remediation strategy and that the patient will follow that recommendation. For the moment, let's assume all of this is correct, and ask whether a visit with a clinician in the first seven days after discharge reduces readmission.

Let's start with a hypothetical experiment. How might an analysis be set up? First, it would be necessary to collect the hospital discharge history of all patients older than age sixty-five. Second, these patients would be divided into two groups—one with and one without an outpatient physician visit within seven days of discharge. Third, the rate of readmissions for those two groups would be reviewed, starting from the moment of discharge and going forward seven days.

An analysis is provided in table 9. What do you see?

Table 9. Cumulative percentage of patients readmitted with and without a doctor visit in the first seven days after discharge

	By Day 3	By Day 5	By Day 7
No doctor visit in first 7 days	3.0% (2.8, 3.2)	4.7% (4.4, 4.9)	6.0% (5.7, 6.3)
Doctor visit in first 7 days	1.6% (1.3, 1.9)	3.2% (2.8, 3.5)	5.2% (4.8, 5.7)

Note: Parentheses include a range of values built by a statistical model.

Of the patients who saw a physician in the first seven days after hospital discharge, only 1.6 percent, were readmitted by day three, as compared to 3.0 percent of those without a doctor visit. The values in parentheses indicate the confidence interval which is range of values built by a statistical model that is consistent with the observed value. The confidence interval gives a sense of how the values might change if the study were to be repeated. To be meaningfully different, the results and their confidence intervals should not overlap. In comparing the confidence interval for day three, readmission percentages between those who saw a doctor (1.3 percent and 1.9 percent) and those who did not (2.8 percent and 3.2 percent), the confidence intervals did not overlap, so the difference was real and did not occur by chance alone.

By day five, 3.2 percent of those with an outpatient visit were readmitted, while those without an outpatient visit had a readmission rate of 4.7 percent. Thus, it would seem that doctor visits after discharge protect patients from readmission—a result you might think is obvious.

But was this study a fair test of the question? There is a word for this sort of analytic error—*tautology*.

This tautology can be stated as, "if you are not readmitted in the first seven days, then you have zero readmissions in the first seven days." This statement sounds quite silly, but consider for a moment what the proposed study asked: If a patient completed an appointment with a doctor in the first seven days after discharge, was the patient readmitted? What is the real implication of the doctor visit in this scenario? The answer is that if a patient was able to keep an outpatient doctor's appointment, then clearly the patient was not in the hospital. The patient cannot be at risk for hospitalization if the logic requires that an appointment be kept that can only take place outside of the hospital itself. If a doctor requires that the patient be seen within the first seven days after discharge, then this guarantees that from discharge time to the kept appointment, it is *structurally impossible* for the patient to be readmitted to the hospital. The study's requirement of a doctor visit is an absolute barrier to readmission until after the doctor visit, hence the tautology.

The reason you cannot recognize a tautology with an outcome of zero admissions is due to the fact that while the patient is required to have the outpatient experience within the first seven days, this hypothesis is looking at readmission from day zero to day seven after discharge, so there is clearly an opportunity for an admission to occur, but only after the patient's first doctor visit. The reduction of readmission risk does not eliminate *all* readmissions, so there is no zero count, which would otherwise alert you to the foolishness of the design.

Now let's consider a new study design without the tautology trap.

Define two groups of patients. Require that both groups must be discharged from the hospital and not readmitted in the first seven days after discharge. One group sees a doctor in the first seven days. The other does not. Both groups are followed from their date of discharge for fourteen days. By definition no one will have an admission in the first seven days. However, from day seven to day fourteen, it is possible to test the utility of the doctor visit in the first seven days after discharge to prevent a readmission in day seven to day fourteen. The results are provided in table 10.

Table 10. Cumulative percentage of patients readmitted with or without doctor visit after first seven days after discharge

	By Day 8	By Day 10	By Day 15
No doctor visit in first 7 days	0.4% (0.2, 0.5)	2.1% (2.0, 2.3)	4.1% (3.9, 4.4)
Doctor visit in first 7 days	1.6% (0.3, 0.4)	2.8% (2.5, 3.2)	5.8% (5.3, 6.2)

Surprisingly, patients who visited their doctors actually had a higher cumulative percentage readmission by days eight, ten, and fifteen. For example, by day fifteen, patients who saw their doctors had a readmission rate of 5.8 percent as compared to 4.1 percent of patients who did not see their doctors.

This is the exact opposite of what we would expect—surprisingly. The results show that a doctor's visit is associated with a higher readmission rate.

Could it be that seeing a doctor puts a patient at greater risk for rehospitalization? If a medical visit is protective, why are there higher readmission rates for those who see their doctors?

Implicit in this confusion is the assumption that both groups of patients—those seen and those not seen by their doctors—are, in fact, comparable at baseline. We make the assumptions that they are equally ill, equally likely to be readmitted prior to a doctor visit, and the post-discharge physician visit is a completely random event and the only relevant factor.

This is, of course, not true. Observational experience is not the same as a randomized controlled trial. Patients are referred to early follow up when they are sicker. Patients themselves aggressively seek follow-up care when they are sicker. Therefore, the fact there is a completed post-discharge follow-up appointment is likely an indication that either the doctor recognized the patient as sicker, or the patient self-identified as sicker and in need of follow-up intervention.

We should therefore not be surprised that patients who are sicker end up readmitted to the hospital faster than patients who are less sick. Freed from the original flawed tautologic design, we fall into the arms of a selection bias for sicker patients.

Incidentally, while it is possible to explain the higher readmission rate while insisting that doctor visits post discharge are effective at reducing hospital readmissions, we must still actually consider the possibility that these visits increase the probability of readmission. In fact, as strange as it may seem, this question is an open controversy.

In 1996 Weinberger et al.[13] initiated a randomized controlled trial to assess the impact of increased primary care access on patients with chronic medical conditions at the Veterans Affairs. In particular, they evaluated the relationship between primary care access and rates of readmission. They found that those assigned to close follow up by a nurse and primary care physician had significantly higher rates of readmission and days of hospitalization than those given usual care.

Consider why this might be the case. First, there is the heretical possibility that a patient who sees a doctor get sicker *because* of the doctor's efforts. Perhaps medications and interventions hurt rather than help.

Perhaps transient clinical deteriorations after hospital discharge are the norm, but if left to themselves, these deteriorations would spontaneously remit. Perhaps doctors and nurses, by aggressively responding to unimportant transient deteriorations, interfere with the natural healing processes.

Perhaps while clinician interventions extend life in the long term, in the short term they challenge patients' homeostasis, which may briefly worsen their conditions, necessitating hospitalization. Under this approach, clinicians trade the short-term worsening and hospitalization of a small subgroup of patients for the clinical benefit of a larger group, achieved after windows of observation of arbitrary duration, such as thirty-day readmissions rather than 180 days.

It is also important to keep in mind that the most important intervention post-discharge might not be clinical. Intervention might take the form of social services, such as a caregiver to pick up medication from the pharmacy, to provide meals, and to compensate for mistakes made in discharge planning.

The purpose of this chapter is not to definitively answer the question of whether seeing a doctor after discharge is beneficial, but rather to sensitize you to the challenges of evaluating observational data and of the need to always be on the lookout for self-imposed tautologies and biases.

5

HEADS OR TAILS—WHICH END IS UP?

Choosing Between Two Sides of a Durational Event

IN DAILY LIFE WE take language for granted, using words and phrases in accustomed ways. We know how to ask questions, get answers, and assimilate those answers so we can act upon that information. This process is so automatic that we think it trivial. But when we seek to communicate in unfamiliar domains, we must confront subtle complexities.

Consider this simple question: What is the readmission rate of patients discharged from a hospital? In asking this question, is the readmission rate for all hospitalizations of a particular patient considered? If a person has been readmitted four times during the year, are all four hospitalizations eligible for the report? Or, is only one discharge per patient counted? If only one hospitalization per patient, then which one should count? The first? The last? A random discharge?

Once it is decided which hospitalization(s) to count, then the point from which to calculate elapsed time until the new hospitalization must be determined. This creates a struggle within the fuzzy notion of hospitalization as an object of durational time.

A hospitalization has two endpoints—a head (start or admission date) and a tail (end or discharge date). Should you count days until readmission from date of admission or from date of discharge of the original hospitalization? If you count from date of admission, then you are counting as elapsed time days that the patient spent in the hospital in the original hospitalization. Do you really believe a patient is at risk for readmission during the initial hospital stay? No, of course not—the patient is already in the hospital. It is only after discharge that a patient is at risk for readmission. Therefore it only makes sense to consider elapsed time until readmission—from date of discharge.

Is everyone discharged from the hospital at risk for readmission? Well, if in the original hospitalization a patient is discharged to the grave (i.e., the person died), this patient poses zero risk for readmission. We can exclude both religiously inspired reports of "resurrection," and the unique 1930s Chicago experience that the dead not only rise, but also vote and vote often! Our experience is that the dead are not at risk for readmission, so we exclude them from our readmission calculations.

Lest you think you are now done with the durational event of hospitalization, there is at least one more consideration.

When using the discharge date for the readmission-rate analytic and excluding the dead, we are functionally ignoring the mortality rate in our original hospital stay. But do we really want to ignore the dead in a global quality metric linked to readmission?

Let's ponder a macabre hypothetical. Consider the implausible, unethical possibility that a medical professional identifies the sickest, most readmission-prone patients during their hospitalizations and consciously kills them. What does this barbaric behavior produce in readmission statistics? By culling the herd of sickest patients, their inclusion is eliminated in the readmission statistic, allowing only the surviving healthy patients to be discharged alive, thereby engineering a low readmission rate!

While no one suspects any hospital of consciously using this horrifying technique to improve its readmission statistics, let's suppose a push for shorter stays with rapid discharges causes hospitals to aggressively institute interventions such as rapidly escalating medication doses to achieve target goals quickly, which compromises those who are the weakest, functionally killing them. While inadvertent, the effect on readmission rates would be the same.

To thwart this extremely perverse incentive for tolerating increased in-hospital mortality by blinding the quality process, medical professionals need to consider an additional quality metric: days from patient's admission to either death or readmission. The start time must be the moment of hospital admission, with the ability to capture all downstream deaths, including those of the index hospitalization itself. Patients upon admission are immediately eligible for death, so it is appropriate to capture elapsed follow-up time from admission to the outcome: death or readmission.

As the trend for public reporting of hospital quality metrics becomes fully established, it will be critical that the chosen metrics do not blindly focus success on one metric at the expense of our very lives.

6

Does My Regional Health Information Organization Prevent Hospital Admissions?

IN MOST LOCALES, PATIENT medical information is trapped in paper records or in the electronic medical record of a single hospital. A patient presenting to a different hospital or emergency room is plain out of luck. Medications, medical tests, and previous surgeries are unavailable to treating physicians at other hospitals, who must rely on patient memory for clinical history—something especially difficult when the patient is unconscious.

A Regional Health Information Organization (RHIO) is an entity created to share medical information, with patient consent, among caregivers from different hospitals. Sharing is designed to improve care and reduce costs. Cost reduction may occur when abnormalities already evaluated elsewhere, which might otherwise drive additional testing or hospital admission, can be safely ignored. Conversely, patients whose history identifies a need for specific care can receive timely intervention.

To justify the funding of these RHIOs, government funders have asked for proof of savings. Leaving aside the obvious answer that information at point-of-care is inherently valuable and is as necessary as washing one's hands before surgery, let's accept the challenge and enter into this conversation.

How is it possible to prove that the existence of a RHIO prevents unnecessary hospital admissions and thus saves money?

Let's assume that the following information is available. There is a list of every patient seen in the ER over a year's time, a record of whether that patient's RHIO record was accessed, and a record of whether that patient was admitted. All diagnoses each patient received in the year prior to the ER visit are also known. Is it possible to deduce from this set of data whether the RHIO prevented admissions?

Consider the design assumptions of this potential study. It might be assumed that accessing the RHIO is independent of any clinical likelihood that a patient will need admission. This assumption means that ER doctors search the RHIO data as often for patients they initially expect to admit as for patients they expect to discharge to home. If we accept this assumption, then it is the information obtained from the RHIO data, and not a biased act of seeking it, that determines whether a patient is admitted. If, on the other hand, it is assumed that doctors look in the RHIO database only when they have already decided that the patient will probably not require admission, then finding that patients for whom doctors sought RHIO information were less often admitted would reflect doctors' choice to use the RHIO, not the impact of the data itself.

In assuming admission equipoise, less frequent admissions of patients for whom doctors sought RHIO data would argue for an RHIO-protective effect against admissions. Of course, it would be necessary to adjust for other known differences—such as number of prior admissions, number of diagnoses, age—but the basic structure of the analysis is straightforward.

We should not expect that every patient for whom a RHIO search was done should have a preventable admission. Some patients will have no data in the RHIO repository. Some of the RHIO data may actually argue for admission. For a small subset of patients, their data history could prevent admission. One would have to first estimate the proportionate size of this group and then allow time to acquire enough emergency department patients to adequately power the study.

The problem with this potential design is its core assumption—the use of the RHIO to obtain medical history is independent of doctors' suspicions of the necessity for admission. In the previous paragraph, adjustment for severity of illness was considered, but it is not possible to adjust for unevenly distributed **unmeasured** indices of severity. What is meant by unmeasured? In any clinical encounter, clinicians believe they get a sense of the patient and the clinical sickliness that is not always quantifiable and therefore not recorded. Analysts have to be concerned that this perception may drive the decision to use the RHIO data system— as illustrated below.

If emergency department doctors, under great pressure to make rapid admission decisions, use the RHIO system only for patients who are less sick to justify their decision not to admit, while patients who obviously require admission do not merit a RHIO review, then it would unfairly appear that the use of the RHIO system is protective against admission. It is possible to suspect this bias by looking at the distribution of **measurable** variables associated with disease severity. If there was more measurable severity in those without a RHIO search, then there might be a concern that there was also an imbalance in the unmeasured variables of severity as well—unmeasured, yes, but perceptible to the emergency department doctor, driving behavior, and unavailable for model adjustment.

Is there an escape from this trap? One escape is just to reject the objection out of hand. Sure, there are unmeasured variables, but they probably vary with the measured ones, so the adjustment of the measured ones is sufficient. Additionally, while it may be true that the information for those less likely to be admitted is disproportionately sought, this information is sought precisely for the reason the RHIO was built in the first place—to find admission-preventive evidence. It is unlikely that without this evidence a patient would have been denied admission or at least denied admission at the same rate. These last statements, while reasonable, are not quantified, and therefore constitute a form of hand waving.

There is a study design that can escape this trap, but it requires a step back to gain a broader perspective. In doing so, more noise will have to be accepted, but in the end inferential integrity will compensate for the noise.

If RHIO functionality is protective against admission, then when RHIO functionality is disrupted, either through unexpected system failure or scheduled downtime for upgrades, admission experience should reflect the impact of this data access loss. By comparing admission rates during these downtimes with the experience when the RHIO is fully operational, the resulting difference should be attributable to the contribution of the RHIO itself.

7

How Could Your Privacy Decisions Impact My RHIO Experience?

Don't Silence My Silence

REGIONAL HEALTH INFORMATION ORGANIZATIONS were created to enable patients to allow their doctors access to all their clinical information from all healthcare institutions at the time and point-of-care. Patients control this process by either opting in or opting out. In the opt-in model, a patient is assumed to have chosen not to participate, and a specific written statement of desire to be included must be obtained before information is shared. In the opt-out model, the assumption is that a patient consents to participate in data sharing, and only those who make a specific effort to opt out later are removed from the process.

In addition to these two models of permission, in the early days of the RHIOs there was talk of allowing patients even greater granularity of control. Some wanted patients to be able to exclude specific information such as drug use, mental illness, or abortions. It is clear that such information loss might compromise an individual's care. Without knowledge of interacting drugs or medical conditions, a treating ER physician could inadvertently make a mistake.

Question: Does your neighbor's ability to censor his or her clinical records impact the meaningfulness of yours?

Answer: Yes. When someone silences his or her medical record, it changes the meaning of the silence in yours. If your medical record does not speak of depression, and if all patients in the RHIO allow all their information to be revealed, then the absence of this history of depression in your medical record is, in fact, meaningful. Your doctors have, by their silence, testified that they do not believe that you are depressed and are not on antidepressant medications. If, however, a participant in the RHIO is allowed the option of silencing any part of his or her record, then the silence in your record is devalued. The silence could be due to suppression of the facts or to the absence of the disease.

It is for this reason that it is not a benign act to give every individual unlimited personal choice. You can opt in or opt out of sharing your entire medical record, but you are not allowed to silence my silence.

Accountability

8

AM I MY BROTHER'S KEEPER?
……...CAIN, SON OF ADAM, TO G-D

The New Longitudinal Healthcare Paradigm

TWO CENTURIES AGO, PATIENTS and physicians shared an episodic notion of medical care. The patient would perceive a medical problem, say a serious laceration, and present to the physician for diagnosis and treatment. Once treatment was delivered, the physician's responsibility was over. It was up to the patient to initiate any subsequent visit. There was no notion of preventive care. There was no notion of surveillance initiated or maintained by a doctor.

Now throughout the United States there are notions of "accountable care" and "medical home." Physicians are accountable for care, and this accountability includes long-term, measurable outcomes, such as control of blood pressure, cholesterol, or diabetes.

As point of fact, it is really the patient and doctor together who share this responsibility.

How should doctors measure the success of their clinics, for example, in controlling blood sugar? First, the measure of interest must be decided. Second, what constitutes success must explicitly be decided.

In diabetes, the hemoglobin A1c test is a good measure of how well the blood sugar has been controlled over time. The lower the hemoglobin A1c, the better diabetes is controlled. Now, how should doctors go about assessing the overall performance of their clinics?

This might seem like an easy challenge. First, choose a threshold hemoglobin A1c value below which diabetes control is considered to be good. Second, monthly determine the percentage of tests below this threshold. If the percentage achieving a value below the threshold is increasing, the patients are doing better; if the percentage is decreasing, the patients are doing worse.

Question: Why does this method look reasonable while actually profoundly misleading?

Answer: Obviously, this metric is subject to manipulation. Suppose there is a group of patients with good diabetes control. To improve performance, a doctor just has to test them more often. Or, if there are patients with bad control, to game the system a doctor could choose not to test them at all or as infrequently as possible. Of course, this sort of premeditated manipulation is unthinkable for an ethical physician.

But, in the real world, we see its functional equivalent.

A decade ago, Montefiore identified patients with extremely poor diabetes control by a hemoglobin A1c greater than 9.5. Note, I am saying patients. We did not count the number of laboratory tests because there might be more than one per patient. We counted each person only once in the year of follow up and used the date of his or her first hemoglobin A1c as the date that defined the patient as an eligible "badly controlled diabetic." Over the course of a year, we found 3,130 patients system-wide with this extremely poor hemoglobin A1c. We then asked ourselves a very simple question: What percentage of these patients had a repeat hemoglobin A1c between six months and twelve months after the initial awful value?

We did not ask who was brought under good control. We only asked who was under active surveillance. The best-practice frequency of testing is on the order of three to four times a year. We discovered that only 1,891 (64 percent) had been retested. This means that 34 percent of these poorly controlled patients would not have contributed to the old-style monthly hemoglobin A1c test surveillance metrics, and were therefore silenced by lack of follow-up testing.

The cohort analysis—following a group of patients to targeted outcome and noticing who has not been seen—is a critical feature of the new philosophy of accountable care and medical home. Cohort analysis can be performed with specialized software, which creates cohorts for follow up and then provides analytic opportunities at different elapsed times for those patients. Institutions without such software create diabetic registries—a list of living diabetic patients—to then assess the success of their diabetic cohort to achieve targeted goals.

A good way to reinforce accountability is to consider all the missing patients as failures. This then highlights the lost patients as well as the need for outreach efforts. Indeed, such a standard affirms commitment to longitudinal care responsibility.

At Montefiore Medical Center, a group of clinicians caring for impoverished homeless patients in the South Bronx accepted the challenge of longitudinal care responsibility. Using our cohort builder and tracking individuals over time, these patients were able to achieve quality outcomes in preventive medicine, which surpassed those achieved in commercially insured populations. They were the first in our organization to achieve national certification as "patient-centered medical home level three"—a significant achievement.

In effect, by dint of commitment to longitudinal care, Montefiore clinicians had created a medical home for the homeless.

9

TO CORRUPT MAN

An Impossible Goal, Inadequate Surveillance, Harsh Punishment, and a Failure of Integrity and Leadership Promote the Dishonorable

AT THE TIME OF my writing of this chapter, a huge scandal surfaced at the Veterans Administration hospitals. A number of deceitful strategies were allegedly employed by VA staff to leave the impression in the electronic medical record that patients were receiving timely appointments.

Under one such manipulation, staff scheduled patients for appointments immediately upon request but purposely did not tell the patients the date of their appointments. Having now documented a timely appointment, the staff canceled the appointment, making it appear that the patient had decided not to accept the appointment. A shadow list was kept to schedule the patient when appointments became available beyond the surveillance capability of the electronic medical record.

In another deception, the VA staff ignored the patient's real date request for an appointment, found the next available appointment, and fraudulently entered the next available date as the patient's chosen date. These two techniques, as well as others, took advantage of the weaknesses of the electronic reporting system, which was designed with the assumption of administrative personal integrity. National VA appointment statistics based on this phony data entry painted a rosy picture of healthcare access with successful administrators paid for performance.

Eric Shinseki, a retired four-star army general wounded in Vietnam, who was serving as the US Secretary of Veteran Affairs at the time of the scandal, was quoted as saying, "I can't explain the lack of integrity among some of the leaders of our healthcare facilities. This is something I rarely encountered during thirty-eight years in uniform. And so I will not defend it, because it is indefensible. But I can take responsibility for it, and I do."[14]

There was no way for the VA patients to enter their own requests for appointments, so there was no permanent record against which scheduled appointments could be compared.

Massive corruption was alleged across multiple facilities. How might this have been prevented?

The *New York Times* stated:

"The seeds of Mr. Shinseki's departure may have been planted years ago, when he established standards that his supporters said were admirable but unrealistically high. He set 125 days as the goal for processing disability claims and was then blamed for the backlog that ensued. For new patients, he required that veterans be seen within two weeks. In the audit, that 14-day standard was singled out as an "organizational leadership failure" and a major problem in providing timely care, second only to a shortage of doctors.[15"]

The *New York Times* claimed that an impossible goal drove the practitioners to corrupt themselves:

"Meeting a 14-day wait-time performance target for new appointments was simply not attainable given the ongoing challenge of finding sufficient provider slots to accommodate a growing demand for services. Imposing this expectation on the field before ascertaining required resources and its ensuing broad promulgation represent an organizational leadership failure."

It may surprise the non-specialist reader, but the immediate recommendation was to relax the performance target.

While a discussion about goals, integrity, and motivation is important to foster a sustainable culture of shared improvement effort, it begs the question that I now pose to the reader.

Question: How could this problem have been detected? What sort of surveillance system could have been put in place that would have made it more difficult to fraudulently claim that care access was achieved? What cohort question could have been used to detect care access inadequacy?

Answer: One possibility would be to track the number of clinic visits completed for each category of patient per year, and develop norms per diagnostic category per year in the different VA facilities, comparing each facility against those norms. The problem, of course is that number of visits does not equate to timeliness of visits, and system-wide access failure would not be detected by using intra-system comparisons.

Another possibility would be to build cohorts of VA patients using unalterable computerized time stamps—such time stamps defeat human manipulation. Elapsed time would be calculated from the moment of appointment request until the date of appointment consummation. Even if the appointment request was cancelled the cancelled appointment request would persist in this analysis and would be used to generate a calculation of elapsed time until the next appointment of the same type.

Profiles of this metric could be built by category of patient and by facility, and then performance among facilities could be compared. Facilities with results that are "too good" or with too little statistical variation would be flagged as potentially fraudulent. Consider the Bernie Madoff stock scandal, in which Madoff claimed consistent earnings year after year—something that is statistically impossible in the stock market.

It would also be possible to build profiles of percentage of visits canceled before the date of the appointment and then compare those across the VA.

A general rule of thumb is that whatever is not monitored is not optimized, and sometimes not even done. Healthcare delivery systems have an affirmative obligation for ongoing surveillance of access and process of care.

Lest anyone believe that somehow such behavior is unique to VA culture, I have two stories that should disabuse you of that notion.

A hospital that shall go unnamed instituted an electronic medication administration system. To make sure that the correct patient was receiving the correct medication, each nurse was required to scan the patient's identity bracelet before giving the medication to confirm that the correct patient had been identified. If performed as designed, with the nurse scanning the patient just before administering medication, the nurse would be warned by the computer if the wrong medication was about to be given to the wrong patient. In this particular hospital, medications were released to the nurses without the bedside scan, so the temporal proximity of scan to medication administration was completely dependent upon the nurses' behavior, not a forced function. A forced function in this case would have locked the medications in the medication cart until a patient's identity bracelet scan released it. For weeks the new process seemed to be working well; that is, because nobody was looking.

When a statistical analysis was done that tracked time from scan to medication administration, an amazing discovery was made. One nurse was effectively scanning patients and administering medication for an entire floor in sixty seconds. Not even The Flash of DC Comics fame could have pulled this off, because even if a nurse could run from bed to bed that quickly, it is not realistic to expect all patients to swallow their medications that fast.

Question: How did this nurse defeat the process?

Answer: She printed out all the armbands for all the patients a second time, administered the medication in her usual way, and scanned the second armbands in the nursing station, followed by an immediate documentation of medication administration. Of course, most nurses did not do this, but the important point is if surveillance is not maintained on some basic level, it is expected that some people will corrupt themselves in unexpected ways.

In a second story, in an experience from early in my career, I set up a database with a force function requiring the entry of a numeric value for the patient identification number before the database would allow additional data entry. I neglected to check the database until six months later, only to find to my horror that while every patient had a number assigned, that number was not a medical record number. Rather it was often just 999999999. Failure to maintain surveillance and failure to provide timely feedback created the foundation for mischief.

10

I Am Not Responsible Until I Say I Am

The Folly of Reliance on Unexamined Billing Processes

MOST PATIENT CARE IN the United States is paid via a fee-for-service model. A healthcare provider renders a service, and for each service submits a bill for reimbursement. By contrast, in the capitated model, the provider is paid a fixed monthly payment for all care, so there is no incentive to provide unnecessary service and no incentive to document details of care.

In the fee-for-service world, billing data is often seen as highly reliable. Given the penalties for fraud, as well as the tradition for personal integrity, healthcare providers do not usually bill for services they have not performed. Given their monetary self-interest in reimbursement, most clinicians will remember to record their activity with a bill. While there are significant limitations to the extent of information available from billing data, its completeness in the fee-for-service world is not questioned.

So what would you say to a home healthcare organization taking its first baby steps assessing its own effectiveness at reducing hospital readmissions? The prevailing wisdom is that the appropriate use of home healthcare can identify and remediate problems in the care of vulnerable patients who, if left to their own devices, would otherwise return to the hospital.

Surprisingly, it turns out that the use of billing data actually gives a pass to home health agencies and makes them look better than they are.

Question: Why is this?

Answer: Consider the sequence of events from the patient's perspective and the flow of responsibility from the perspective of the home health organization.

A patient is to be discharged from a hospital. Let's assume that the patient needs home healthcare and is referred to a home health agency, but due to staff shortages or precipitous discharge to meet hospital length-of-stay quality targets, no one from the agency can perform an evaluation in the hospital before discharge. The patient is seen at home by the home health agency on day two or day three after discharge, when appropriate care is provided. The home healthcare agency dates its bill two or three days post discharge, and this patient is included among the number of patient's at risk for readmission in the service's thirty-day readmission summary report.

What is terribly wrong with this picture? For vulnerable home health patients, care in the first two days after hospital discharge is crucial, and readmissions in this window before they are even seen by the home health care agency a serious failure. Allowing the home healthcare bill to determine the time of onset of responsibility, functionally discounts any hospital readmission in the first two to three days post discharge—the days of highest risk. Further, after ridding itself of these pesky sickly patients in the first two days, the readmission metric now has the audacity to not only count the healthier people but also to attribute to each of them thirty days of follow up risk days when in fact they only had risk for 28 days.

What should happen is that the home healthcare agency should take responsibility prior to discharge—actually, from the moment of referral. Any metric of adequacy of care would have to include all the hospital-discharged patients referred to them, not just those they saw. Failure to make that initial contact in the first day back home, and any subsequent admission prior to a billable event, would not immunize the agency against accountability for that readmission. That readmission should be included in the agency's statistics.

11

WHO IS RESPONSIBLE FOR THE EVENTS OF THE HOSPITALIZATION?

A COLLEAGUE ASKED ME to identify the field in Montefiore's information system designating the physician responsible for a patient's care during a hospitalization. He was interested in creating performance reports for dashboards and report cards, and wanted to attribute these outcomes to a single physician who could be held accountable. My answer to him was that his question was more philosophical than lexical.

Question: What do you think is the problem with this question? Is there an answer to it?

Answer: On some level, you feel there must be a responsible, identifiable party. However, the problem is not that I do not have an answer—the problem is that the question is inadequately defined.

Consider two scenarios for which responsibility could be sought:

Scenario #1

Upon discharge from the hospital, a patient is sent home with drugs that interact with each other, compromising the effectiveness of both. On the day of discharge, the medication set is not evaluated for interactions.

Scenario #2

On day 4 of a hospitalization, a patient cannot be discharged because the home environment is not safe for the patient's level of function. This level of function was known at the time of admission, and there was no reasonable expectation of improvement during the hospitalization. No social worker had been engaged at the start of admission to assess options.

Clearly, the medication problem in the first example is only knowable on the day of discharge, and is the responsibility of the discharge physician. With the second example, the home safety issue should have been knowable on admission. The admitting physician should have considered the need for a social service consult, and the resulting elongated length of stay is the admitting physician's responsibility.

Attribution of responsibility is task and target specific and does not allow for "one person responsible for all." Care coordination is especially complex in an era of many physicians managing a patient—admitting, discharge, night call, and daytime hospitalists. In addition, there may be many services involved in a patient's care—surgery, medicine, and rehabilitation. The solution to the complex processing of a patient and preparation for subsequent discharge is a system-wide responsibility, not a single person globally responsible for all failures. Designing a system to create checklists, monitor processes, and fix mistakes to inform the process of managing the next patient is the challenge of our age.

Data Analytics and Predictive Models

12

Epidemic of Diastolic Dysfunction in the Bronx

Knowing the Source is Half the Battle

A MEDICAL RESIDENT CAME by my office after noticing something odd when using our patient cohort builder, Clinical Looking Glass. He discovered that Montefiore had suffered an extraordinary epidemic of diastolic dysfunction congestive heart failure between 2005 and 2007.

Diastolic dysfunction congestive heart failure is a disease that resembles congestive heart failure, with shortness of breath and leg swelling, but there is a normal heart pumping function when the heart is studied with an echocardiogram. The cause of this disease is the inability of the heart to relax between pumps of blood, often a result of thickened walls due to the damaging effect of chronic high blood pressure. The unrelaxed heart backs up blood to the lungs, causing shortness of breath, and backs up blood to the rest of the body, causing lower leg swelling (edema).

Table 11 summarizes our resident's observations.

Table 11. Diagnosis of diastolic congestive heart failure by year at Montefiore Medical Center

Year	Number of patients with diastolic CHF	Percentage increase from preceding year
2005	170	–
2006	308	+81%
2007	531	+72%

As you can see, from 2005 to 2006, the number of patients with diastolic dysfunction CHF increased by 138 (81 percent). From 2006 to 2007, the number increased by 223 (72 percent).

These increases were certainly dramatic and suspicious for an unrecognized epidemic.

Question: Why do you think we experienced such a huge increase in patients with this disease? Was the actual number of cases increasing, or had the reporting threshold changed?

Answer: Suspicious that this "epidemic" was artificial, we looked at the number of all-cause congestive heart failure patients and the percentage change from year to year. If the diastolic CHF "epidemic" were real, we would expect to see an increase in all-cause CHF patients by the amount increase in diastolic dysfunction. If the "epidemic" was merely a recoding of patients within the general category of congestive heart failure, then we should expect that the all-cause congestive heart failure counts should be stable from year to year.

Our information system codes congestive heart failure with eight distinct categories:

> 428.30 - Unspecified Diastolic Heart Failure
> 428.31 – Acute Diastolic Heart Failure

428.32 – Chronic Diastolic Heart Failure
428.33 – Acute on Chronic Diastolic Heart Failure
428.40 – Unspecified Combined Systolic and Diastolic Heart Failure
428.41 – Acute Combined Systolic and Diastolic Heart Failure
428.42 – Chronic Combined Systolic and Diasatolic Heart Failure
428.43 – Acute on Chronic Combined Systolic And Diastolic

Table 12 shows the changes in percentage and number of patients with diastolic and all-cause congestive heart failure over a three-year period.

Table 12. Diastolic and nonspecific congestive heart failure, Montefiore Medical Center

Year	Number with diastolic CHF	Diastolic dysfunction percentage increase from preceding year	Number with all cause CHF	All cause CHF percentage increase from preceding year
2005	170	Baseline	6,114	Baseline
2006	308	+81%	6,048	-1%
2007	531	+72%	5,957	-2%

Between the years 2005 and 2006, we saw an increase of 81 percent in patients with the diagnosis of diastolic dysfunction type of congestive heart failure. During the same period of time, we saw that all causes of congestive heart failure actually experienced a decline of 1 percent. If this had been a true epidemic of a new disease, we should have expected that the number of patients in the category of all cause congestive heart failure would have increased by 138 cases (308-170). This increase on the base number of all congestive heart failure cases in 2005 (6,114) should have resulted in an increase of 2.2 percent in cases. Instead we saw a 1 percent decline.

In the absence of the expected increase, we have to presume that what we experienced was not an increase in a specific type of congestive heart failure but rather a recoding of some of the other categories of congestive heart failure.

Over the years, Medicare reimbursement policies have changed. Hospitals are now paid considerably more when they provide greater diagnostic specificity. Diastolic or systolic congestive heart failure as a billing diagnosis pays a great deal more than a billing code with nonspecific congestive heart failure. Thus, hospitals have been incentivized to code with greater specificity with the resulting "epidemic" of diastolic congestive heart failure.

This chapter demonstrates the danger of repurposing data without considering its initial purpose. Every data collection serves its primary mission and continues to do so, even as we try to repurpose it. Ignoring its original purpose is done at our peril.

13

Predictive Analytic Surprise

How Good Care Confounds Biologic Intuition in Building Predictive Models

FOR THE LAST FIFTEEN years, the Care Management Organization at the Montefiore Medical Center has focused on a capitated model of accountable care. In return for a fixed monthly payment, Montefiore provides all conventional inpatient and outpatient medical care and a suite of additional services, including post discharge interventions for diabetes and congestive heart failure, calling patients on the phone post discharge to make sure their medications are correct and understood, and referring patients to pharmacists if there are any concerns.

To efficiently use scarce resources, the care management organization decided to develop a predictive analytic to stratify patients by risk of readmission and to prioritize follow-up care for those at highest risk. Montefiore had been using a purchased predictive analytic tool, but it was not based on local experience, nor was it informed by the rich clinical information available to us from our electronic medical records.

Internally, we developed a process to test contenders for the institution's predictive analytic. All new models vied with one another for dominance. New models were built on a training data set and then competed with the commercial model on a completely new data set. The observed thirty-day readmission rate was compared to the predicted rate with the best model chosen for implementation.

The winning model now runs every night at our medical center, using Clinical Looking Glass to identify all the day's discharges. It pulls clinical and administrative data; calculates patients' readmission probabilities; and assigns priorities in work lists for use by the nurses, who make follow-up calls.

This chapter is written because of an unexpected finding.

When we started building the model, we discovered certain clinical information was quite helpful. For example, a previous hospitalization increased the likelihood of a readmission. Male gender (the real weaker sex, as I like to say) was also predictive of increasing admissions. What struck us as surprising, however, was a particular variable that made no biologic sense: a diagnosis of HIV reduced the likelihood of a thirty-day readmission.

Now, HIV, the human immunodeficiency virus, is obviously recognized as a biologically important variable, and it should predict increased readmissions as this virus attacks the immune system and makes a patient vulnerable to infections and cancers.

However, our modeling revealed that an HIV diagnosis—in our hospital in the twenty-first century—was actually protective against readmission.

HIV made its appearance in the 1980s as AIDS, and it was at that time uniformly fatal; it was responsible for one out of every three hospitalizations in some hospitals.

Question: Why in 2015 should such a dangerous disease actually be protective against readmission in our hospital?

Answer: While such a finding seems paradoxical, the answer is quite simple. For years our institution focused on HIV; built excellent follow-up programs; educated our primary care doctors; and staffed our clinics with social workers, nurse practitioners, and infectious disease doctors committed to extending quality of life in patients with this disease. Our predictive model was telling us that our success in managing HIV made it a bad predictor of increased hospital readmission.

This observation made us realize that over time we should expect our predictive models to become progressively less predictive, and we will be tempted to adjust them as our interventions become progressively more successful.

But we should be careful not to ignore the signals of the old models, even as we attempt to refine our models to improve their predictive ability. Remember, the interventions directed by the original model succeeded in reducing readmissions by identifying specific groups for intervention post discharge. Unless we successfully identify and correct the root causes of the problems that require post discharge remediation, the clinical need for post discharge remediation continues to exist. Replacing the model functionally silences it from advising us to continue our efforts in the very population with whom our interventions yielded a positive outcome. This courts disaster because it tells us that those groups no longer need intervention, - a highly suspect assumption.

Understanding what interventions worked and with whom, and correcting root causes requiring remediation in hospital or in discharge planning, are critical goals before mindlessly switching to a new model based on changing predictive performance.

14

Can We Learn from One Another?

Do We Have to Validate Each Study in Our Own Environment?

IN THE PAST, EVIDENCE-BASED medicine advanced with the following paradigm. Small groups of researchers identified a clinical problem, developed a solution, demonstrated its efficacy in a trial, and published the results. Other practitioners read the studies in reputable journals, relied upon those recommended and proven therapies or interventions, and used them in their own population without revalidating locally. This process of evidence-based medicine is considered good practice. There is no need to prove clinical interventions locally before adopting them. Note that this broad description is actually an overstatement—one should always evaluate local effectiveness—but it serves as a convenient foil to my educational purpose.

This accepted standard pattern of behavior has led to an expectation that all things learned elsewhere in an appropriately sized trial with similar patients can be generalized to everywhere without additional local effort.

Question: Is it possible to carry this model of elsewhere-derived confidence into the science of administrative healthcare delivery? Are there some caveats to the automatic acceptance of administrative results discovered in other institutions? What are the implications for predictive models built in different healthcare delivery systems? Can the equations from another institution be carried over without validating them in your own institution?

Answer: In the previous chapters, I noted some important caveats. Another important one here is that categories have meaning dependent upon their institutional and time context.

On the administrative data, this can be easily understood. As institutions engage in efforts to obtain full monetary value for their service delivery through coding optimization, the codes themselves take on different meanings. Changes in national policies for reimbursement over the last decade have espoused dramatic shifts in diagnostic specificity (as seen in the earlier section covering diastolic dysfunction versus nonspecific congestive heart failure), and that specificity is rewarded financially. While the underlying clinical reality does not change, its phenotypic manifestation in coding does.

Between institutions, different clinical interventional efforts on a population health basis will often change the meaningfulness of a diagnostic category. In an institution with no invested effort in managing a particular population of patients, that population may have a high readmission rate, and the diagnoses linked to that population will be strong predictors of readmission. In another institution with a deep commitment to intervention in that diagnostic entity, the diagnosis would paradoxically be protective against readmission. We have seen this in Montefiore's predictive efforts.

In addition, as an institution's interventions are implemented, the meaningfulness of those predictive categories shift as the intervention becomes successful. Therefore, local model modification in the living organism of population health should be ongoing. Healthcare service delivery models are based upon conditions that have local definitional idiosyncrasies embedded within them.

The creation of local models built on temporally enriched cohorts capturing local reality, is critical for ongoing management of populations. While we can certainly learn from one another, we should also realize that just as all politics are local, clinical need, prediction, and surveillance have local color that requires local analytic technology, insight, and ongoing effort.

That is why at Montefiore, local cohort building is an ongoing project.[8]

Our website, Clinical Looking Glass (http:\exploreclg.montefiore.org) describes this activity in greater detail.

15

Adjustment or Excuse?

What Happens When You Adjust for Race?

STATISTICAL MODELS HAVE BECOME much easier to build since the advent of the personal computer. Interpretation, however, still requires judgment.

Question: If you build a model looking at readmission outcomes and you wish to compare the performance of different organizations, which variables should you include? What is the meaning of including a variable **to adjust**?

Answer: Adjustment is usually understood as making sure the comparison is fair—that the differences between hospitals are a consequence of their operational characteristics under their administrative control and not due to variables that are exogenous to the quality of care they provide.

For example, if post discharge readmission rates are used as an indicator of quality comparison between hospitals, obvious no-fault readmissions should be excluded, such as unrelated car accidents or baby deliveries. But, should there be adjustment for race?

To put my biases on the table, I should state at the outset that I find the concept of race distasteful. It has its origin in pseudoscience and as a construct was an abettor of appalling human behavior—the implementation of grotesque notions of eugenics. However, race is often used in modeling.

Let's consider how it might be used. Race could be used to see whether it is a variable that "explains" some variability. If it is noted that certain populations fare worse than others, this could be a signal that work needs to be focused on those communities. This would be a potentially appropriate use of race as a social construct, as it looks at inequities of care or special challenges faced by select groups.

If, however, an institution "adjusts for race" in a self-assessment of the quality of care it provides, then functionally it is giving itself a pass to provide substandard care to its minority populations. This adjustment conceals the failure of such institutions to achieve national goals. If race must be used, use it as a probe to detect potential inequities or special challenges that need to be met, not as an excuse for poor performance.

16

Why Am I Doing Better than You in Each of My Subgroups, but Overall You Are Looking Better than Me?

Simpson's Paradox

IN ONE ANALYSIS I reviewed, I noticed a cost comparison between two institutions. Care provided by Institution A was more expensive per patient than by Institution B. However, when I divided the populations of both institutions into two substrata—patients who died during one year and those who survived the year—Institution A was surprisingly cheaper than Institution B in both strata.

Question: Do you believe this is possible? If so, which metric should a doctor choose to determine where to send patients?

Answer: First, here's a concrete example to show that this phenomenon is indeed possible. I built an example with institutional strata cost values, number of members per strata, and the average cost within each institution that ignores the strata. For each category (stratum) of patient, Institution B is more expensive than Institution A. Table 13 shows the cost per year per patient (survived or died) at both institutions.

Table 13. Cost per patient by institution for those who survived or died in one year

Category of patient	Institution A	Institution B
Survived the year	$100 per patient	$150 per patient
Died during the year	$1,000 per patient	$1,500 per patient

Patients who survived the year cost only $100 per patient at Institution A as compared to the more expensive $150 per patient at Institution B. Patients who died at Institution A cost $1,000 as compared to the higher cost of $1,500 per patient at Institution B.

Table 14 looks at the number of patients in each category at both institutions.

Table 14. Number of patients per category

Category of patient	Institution A	Institution B
Survived the year	100	110
Died during the year	20	5

When the calculated average cost for managing the 120 patients in Institution A is compared to the average cost of the 115 patients in Institution B, we find:

- The average cost per patient at Institution A is (100*$100+20*$1,000)/120 = $250 per person.
- The average cost per patient at Institution B is (110*$150+5*$1,500)/115 = $209 per person.

- For each category of patient, Institution B is more expensive than Institution A ($150>$100 and $1,500>$1,000).
- The average cost per person is the reverse - Institution A is more expensive than Institution B ($250>$209).

The reason behind the final bullet point is pretty simple: patients are always more expensive when they die. Twenty-six percent of all annual Medicare expenses are attributable to care for patients in the last year of life.[16] Institution A had a larger proportion of patients in their last year of life as compared to Institution B (20 out of 120 versus 5 out of 115), so the overall average cost sampled more from the category of last year of life and was therefore more expensive. This is a classic example of Simpson's paradox, where by oversampling a higher attack rate stratum, you end up with a higher overall rate.

A plausible explanation for why proportionately more people are dying in Institution A than in Institution B might be that Institution A cares for much older patients, and thus the death rate itself is not a cause for concern.

To find the cost effective institution for a patient referral, the doctor must identify clinically cogent strata and make the comparison in the stratum relevant to his patient.

Developing Longitudinal Intuition

17

Does Zero Mean Never?

How the Question, Its Context, and Statistics Drive Judgment

IMAGINE THE FOLLOWING CLINICAL scenario: a patient walks into an emergency room complaining of chest pain. The pain completely resolves while being evaluated in the ER. How likely is this chest pain due to a rare condition of slow tearing of the aorta with the threat of a ruptured aortic aneurysm?

The aorta is the major blood highway from the heart, bringing blood to all parts of the body. It is basically a tube that, in the case of an aortic aneurysm, becomes damaged and bulges like a balloon. If the walls of this blood vessel begin to tear, the patient feels significant pain, and without surgical repair, the tear can proceed to rupture, causing internal bleeding and death. The tear can be detected through the use of a CT scan to visualize the aorta, but this involves radiation exposure.

A ruptured aortic aneurysm is rare, so strategies to reduce unnecessary radiation exposure have been considered.

Question: If you're a doctor, how might you approach this problem?

Answer: The first step is to look at the experience of patients with these constellations of symptoms in your own hospital.

At Montefiore, a group of clinicians reviewing the charts of patients suspected of having this critical condition found that of the nineteen patients whose pain completely resolved in the ER prior to undergoing a diagnostic CT scan, none had evidence on the CT scan of an aortic aneurysm.

Does this zero event in nineteen observations mean that, in the future, if a patient's pain resolves, our hospital should never expect to see an aortic aneurysm? If not never, what is the highest possible probability of finding an aortic aneurysm consistent with this experience?

Given this experience, if another patient came into the emergency room with chest pain that fully resolved, should a doctor feel comfortable stopping all further evaluation?

Let's develop our intuition by building a hypothetical model.

Suppose you asked G-d for the real risk of an aortic aneurysm, and you were told that the risk was 17 percent. How often might you expect to see nineteen patients in a row without an aortic aneurysm?

Imagine red and white balls. The red balls represent patients with aortic aneurysms and the white balls represent healthy patients. Place seventeen red balls (diseased patients) and eighty-three white balls (healthy patients) in a bag. Shake the bag, blindly draw a ball, and record its color. Put the chosen ball back into the bag, shake the bag, draw out another ball, and record its color. Repeat this procedure nineteen times and ask: Were any of the balls red? If not, record this series of nineteen draws as evidence of no disease. This would be a sample of nineteen white balls and zero red balls—zero events.

Repeat the experiment of nineteen draws one thousand times and record the percentage of time you find no disease. This percentage is a measure of consistency of 17 percent (seventeen red balls in one hundred balls), with our experience of zero observations in nineteen trials.

You can do this with an actual bag of balls or perform a computer simulation!

In my simulations, I found that when the true rate of disease is 17 percent, you can expect to see nineteen draws of zero 2.8 percent of the time.

This means that the previous observation of zero events in nineteen patients is consistent 2.8 percent of the time, with a true rate of disease of 17 percent. A doctor would now have to make a judgment call. If a possible disease rate is consistent with observable reality only 2.8 percent of the time, is that consistent enough to make the associated hypothesized 17% risk of disease the risk to use in clinical decision making. To justify the expense and radiation exposure of CT testing should we be using the possibility of 17% risk of disease in our considerations of risk and benefit?

Conventionally, the research world has considered a probability of less than 2.5 percent to be rare enough to be ignored, so formally 2.8% is not ignorable. Following that logic any clinical decision not to proceed with diagnostic CT must withstand the credible possibility that the risk of aortic aneurysm could be as high as 17%.

There is no absolute rule, so considerations of risk and benefit should be incorporated in the decision.

Following this general framework, table 15 demonstrates how often to expect to see zero of nineteen if the true risk is 1 percent, 5 percent, 10 percent, and 18 percent.

Table 15. True risk versus probability of zero events in nineteen patients

Risk versus probability	Percentage			
True risk of disease	1%	5%	10%	18%
Probability of seeing zero events in 19 patients	83%	37.8%	13.4%	2.2%

Note that if the true risk of disease is 1 percent, it is expected that there would be no disease in nineteen patients 83 percent of time. When the true rate is 5 percent, we would expect to see nineteen zeros in a row 37.8 percent of the time. As the true disease rate goes up, the probability of seeing zero observations nineteen times in a row goes down. If you believe that a true risk of 10 percent is too high to stop testing for this condition, then the associated **13.4 percent** probability of zero events in nineteen patients (which is greater than the conventional **ignorability cutoff of 2.5%**) makes it imperative to continue testing.

From a decision-making perspective, if a doctor feels that the disease is serious enough to warrant the expenditure and radiation risk, even if the disease frequency is 1 percent, then the zero of nineteen, which is consistent 83 percent of the time with a real rate of 1 percent, would also require additional tests to rule out this dangerous disease, even if it means additional radiation exposure.

As I explained above, standard scientific convention considers probabilities of less than 2.5 percent so low as not likely and therefore not consistent with the posited rate of disease. This means that any consistency rate greater than 2.5 percent has an associated disease attack rate that must be considered in any policy decision. Therefore 1 percent, 5 percent, 10 percent, and 17 percent are all consistent with zero of nineteen, and if you would be willing to expose people to monetary cost and radiation risk at any of these four rates of disease, then the finding of zero of nineteen does not allow you to stop.

Turning this question around, suppose a doctor would be satisfied to stop further evaluation if the true risk of disease were 0.001 (1/1,000). How many patients in a row would he have to study with only zero events before deciding the observation was so rarely consistent (0.025) that it must be rarer than 1/1,000?

First recognize that a risk of disease of 1/1,000 means that each patient has a chance of no disease of 999/1,000 = 0.999.

Does Zero Mean Never? | 83

How many no-disease patients would a doctor have to see to be just barely consistent (2.5% of the time) with an expected disease rate of 1/1,000?

For those who remember logarithms from high school, this is easily calculated.

$$0.999^x = 0.025$$

$$\log(0.999^x) = \log(0.025)$$

$$x * \log(0.999) = \log(0.025)$$

$$x = \frac{\log(0.025)}{\log(0.999)}$$

$$x = 3{,}687$$

3,687 zeros in a row is consistent 2.5% of the time with an expected rate of disease of 1/1000. At the 3,688th non-diseased patient in the series you cross the decision threshold. The probability is less than 2.5% consistent; and you could safely say that the true risk of disease is less than 1/1000. Since your decision to continue CT scan workup was predicated on a rate of disease of 1/1000, the absence of disease in the 3,688th patient means you could stop your routine workups.

For those who wish to simulate the example in the freeware of R, the following is provided.

For Those Mathematically and *R*-Programming Inclined (Otherwise Skip)

R simulation uses the following function:
User enters
x = the number of black balls representing the number of patients with disease; y = the number of total balls representing all the patients evaluated, so that x/y represents the "true rate" of disease.
n = the number of times to run the nineteen experiments. The default is 5, but usually 1,000 is entered. The more times the experiment is run of size 19, the more stable the estimate will be of what the outer limits ought to be for the confidence intervals.

Function:
probability of never<–function(x,y,n = 5){
r<–c(rep(1,x), rep(0,($y-x$)))
m<–sample(r,19*y*n, replace = TRUE)
mm<–matrix(m, nrow = y*n)
mmm<–apply(mm,1, sum)
print(sum(as.numeric(mmm<1))/(y*n))
}

Interpretation of the function:

1. Create a vector representing the simulated universe made up of x ones and $y-x$ zeros. If trying to simulate a true reality of 176 per 1,000, enter x = 176 and y = 1,000. This creates a vector of numbers containing 176 ones and 1,000-176, or 824 zeros. The vector would look like this:
    1,1,1,1,......0,0,0...
    (176 ones) (824 zeros).
2. The vector can be thought of as a bag from which is randomly drawn a single value. Record the value, put the value back into the bag, and then randomly draw again. Repeat this process 19*y*n times.

3. Take this vector with its 19*y*n elements and put it into the shape of a matrix with y*n rows. This creates a matrix of y*n rows and 19 columns. Thus, each row has 19 members of zero, or one drawn from the original universe.
4. For each row, sum the values of the row. Since there are 19 values of either 0 or 1, the highest value this sum could have is 19 and the smallest is 0.
5. Test whether the sum of each row is <1. If the sum of a row is <1, that is, equal to zero, this means that this simulated experiment of 19 draws yielded an experiment with zero occurrences. Each zero occurrence experiment is given a numeric truth value of 1. The as numeric command converts this truth value to an integer value of 1. By summing the number of experiments composed of 19 observations with zero events, you are functionally counting the number of the experiments that saw no event. Divide this number by the number of experiments (y*n) to find the simulated probability of no events. This is the probability of no events from a universe with a true rate of x/y.

>probability of never (176,1000,1000)
[1] 0.025392

> Comment: This result is greater than the 2.5th percentile, implying that a value of zero could be consistent with a true rate of 176/1000.

>probability.of.never (177,1000,1000)
[1] 0.024656

> Comment: This result is less than the 2.5th percentile, implying that a value of zero could not be consistent with a true rate of 177/100.

A faster way to get the result is to use a prepared R function from the R Library PropCIs (download from Cran R; http://cran.r-project.org/). PropCIs library is an implementation in R of the article by Clopper and Pearson.[17]

> exactci (0,19,.95)
data:

95 percent confidence interval:
0.0000000 0.1764669

Exact CI shows us that the largest rate that will yield zero result in 19 trials consistent with our notion of 95 percent of its distribution is 0.1764, or 176.4 per 1,000. When you enter the next higher integer value greater than 176.4, which is 177 in our R function "probability.of.never," you find that the probability of zero in 19 consecutive trials occurs at the 0.024656 percentile. This is smaller than the 2.5th percentile, the conventional arbiter of what is considered likely. Therefore, 0 of 19 observations refutes the possibility of a rate as low as 177 per thousand but does not refute the possibility of a rate of 176 per thousand.

18

Will I Be Able to Play the Piano?

Worse Disease Gets Better Outcome
Cull the Herd and Leave Only the Strong

RECENTLY A MEDICAL RESIDENT told me an interesting fact: "Did you know that patients followed for three months after suffering fulminant myocarditis have better ejection fractions than patients with less severe myocarditis?"

The ejection fraction is a measure of how well the heart is able to pump blood. With increasing damage to the heart muscle, the ability of the heart to pump blood is reduced, and the ejection fraction as evaluated on a cardiac echo is similarly reduced.

Fulminant myocarditis is just as it sounds: a rip-roaring inflammation of the heart muscle. Common sense would lead us to conclude that "severe" inflammation should cause greater damage than "mild or moderate" inflammation. Yet, if the resident is correct, the reverse is true. Follow-up post discharge reveals that those with mild or moderate myocarditis have worse heart function than those with much more severe inflammation of the heart muscle.

Question: Why is this?

Answer: When I heard the resident's question, I was immediately reminded of a joke. A skier had a terrible accident and broke his hand. Fortunately, nearby was an excellent orthopedic hospital with one of the world's foremost hand surgeons. The surgery was long and involved, but technically successful.

Upon awakening from anesthesia, the patient asked the surgeon, "How did it go?"

The surgeon reassured him, telling the skier that in a few months he would be as good as new.

The skier asked, "Will I be able to play the piano?"

The surgeon answered, "Yes."

That is great," the skier said. "I didn't know how to play it before."

As this joke implies, context is critical. In the context of a skilled piano player who suffers a skiing accident, the healing would restore hand functionality so the inherent piano playing skill could be manifest in performance. In the context of someone who does not play the piano, the healing would not result in the automatic acquisition of new piano-playing skills!

In the fulminant myocarditis example, the context of the disease and the context of its evaluation are critical to resolving the paradox.

Suppose there are two population of patients—one with baseline mild cardiac damage from whatever cause (previous heart attack, high blood pressure, etc.) and another with serious prior cardiac damage with very low ejection fractions (less than 35).

Now superimpose on these two populations a case of fulminant myocarditis. The patients whose baseline is already severely compromised will probably die and not be available for follow-up evaluation. Those with mild baseline disease will probably become really sick but will survive to be evaluated later. This is an example of survivor bias.

As a result, fulminant myocarditis kills off those with severe heart disease, leaving only those with mild disease to be evaluated later, while mild myocarditis permits those with horrendous heart pump failure at baseline to survive.

If the myocarditis itself leaves no permanent heart damage, then death at the time of the myocarditis culls the patient cohort of its sickest members, leaving only the healthier ones to manifest their relatively good ejection fraction. Thus is explained the paradox of the "worse illness resulting in better outcome."

19

Paradoxical Worsening of Metrics as Care Innovation and Implementation Improves Quality

A Cautionary Tale in Deep Venous Thrombosis

A COLLEAGUE OF MINE made an observation that puzzled him. Over the last ten years, the management of clots in the legs (deep venous thrombosis; DVT) has evolved. New oral agents require fewer lab tests for control of the required blood-thinning maintenance. Intravenous therapy that previously required multiple daily infusions has been dramatically reduced in frequency, making it possible to manage many patients with home intravenous therapy.

These advances have made it obvious that metrics of care quality, such as the length of a hospital stay, should dramatically improve as the need for long hospitalization is reduced. Yet, my colleague's analysis revealed that at his hospital, instead of going down, length of stay had actually gone up.

Question: How is it possible that, despite improving medications and therapies length of hospital stays could actually increase?

Answer: The key solution to this conundrum is recognizing the nature of the metric—length of stay. Length of stay is a measure of the average length of stay for those who have been **admitted** to the hospital.

In the old days, all patients with DVT, with or without serious comorbidities, were admitted for intravenous heparin therapy. Nowadays, selected (read: "healthier") patients can be treated at home with home intravenous therapy, thus precluding admissions. This means that the patients who do traverse the hospital gate and are admitted tend to be sicker than the cohort of DVT patients admitted in the past. The healthier, non-admitted patients should, in fairness, contribute a length of stay of zero to the calculation, thus allowing the quality metric to realize the phenomenal success of preventing these admissions. Unfortunately, the length-of-stay metric only considers those who are admitted into the hospital, and fails to add a zero value for the length of stay of the non-admitted patient in the numerator and an extra patient in the denominator for its calculation. As the only people who are admitted are the sicker patients, their comorbidities drive longer lengths of stay and elongate the length-of-stay measure.

The clinical success and efficiency of my colleague's hospital in coordinating home care utilizing the latest in medical therapies had ironically worsened a prevalent metric of quality, leaving an unfair impression of worsening efficiency.

20

But it Makes Biologic Sense...

The Illusion of the Known: "It isn't what we don't know that gives us trouble. It's what we know that ain't so."—Will Rogers

ONE OF THE GREAT intellectual traps is the illusion of the known. As biologic knowledge produces demonstrable successes, clinicians have become progressively more certain that our intellectual constructs are correct and do not require empiric validation. Smug certainty interferes with the acquisition of knowledge.

Let me take you back to Vienna in the early 1800s. At the time, pregnant women admitted to the hospital to give birth on the medical service died in childbirth at the appalling rate of 10 percent. One in ten healthy women who came to deliver her child was instead delivered to the grave. The cause was unknown, but many "known" things got in the way of progress. One physician, Ignaz Semmelweis, noted that a colleague of his, while performing an autopsy on a woman who had died of puerperal sepsis, was cut on his hand by a student. His wound was contaminated with material from the dead women's infected uterus. The injured physician died within twenty-four hours of what we would recognize today as septicemia—overwhelming infection.

Today we would also easily recognize the common element. The bacterium that had infected the woman's uterus, ultimately killing her, was transmitted through the injury to the hand to the physician, who died of overwhelming infection. However, in Semmelweis's time, it was thought impossible for a male professor of medicine to die from an injury sustained from a dead woman.

Question: Any idea what biologic construct precluded the transmission of disease as we understand it today?

Answer: In Semmelweis's time, all disease was structure-based and identity was inextricably linked to the specific organ and tissue affected. The woman died of a disease in the uterus. Since only a uterine disease was present, a male physician, who by virtue of gender did not have a uterus, could not have died from that which killed the woman. Biologic plausibility in the early 1800s linked the disease to the biologic structure in which it was found. To us, this seems foolish, but medical constructs seem very real in their time. It should also be noted that another "known" fact at that time was that physicians healed through physical contact. It was inconceivable that something about a physician's touch (today's construct of germs) could possibly be the source of the deadly epidemic of women dying in childbirth, which was exactly the case.

You should know that ultimately Semmelweis recognized an empiric relationship between contact with non–organ specific "putrid particles" at autopsy and the onset of disease caused by physicians who moved freely between the autopsy room and the delivery room. By instituting a regimen of chlorine hand washing, Semmelweis dramatically reduced the rate of puerperal sepsis. Unfortunately, the story ends badly for Semmelweis. In his lifetime, the truth of his observations and his empiric successes—repeated multiple times in multiple hospitals—were rejected by his contemporaries. So powerful are medical memes.

You may think this only happened in the distant past, but every generation marinates in its intellectual delusions. In my early years of medical training, it was "known" that abnormal heart rhythms seen around the time of a heart attack were causal of early mortality from arrhythmias. Medications were developed to suppress these abnormal beats. So certain was the medical fraternity that suppression of these beats could only be a good thing that they built their study to demonstrate effectiveness[18] with statistical tests that assumed only the possibility of benefit—not harm. This is known as a one-sided test. Its advantage is that it requires fewer patients in a study, which consequently costs less. It has the disadvantage, however, of reducing the power of a study to detect the supposedly impossible harm caused by the drug, should it exist. As it turned out, the drugs encainide and flecainide were, in fact, dangerous and increased mortality, which through the grace of providence were fortunately detected despite our medical obliviousness.

I remember as a medical student getting into a heated disagreement with my resident about antiarrhythmic drugs—not a particularly bright thing to do when your evaluation is dependent upon your resident's goodwill. He insisted that antiarrhythmics wiped out arrhythmias and were beneficial, but I doggedly insisted that so-called antiarrhythmic drugs were really "heart-state altering agents" whose ultimate benefit had to be proven. My construct turned out to be correct...this time. But no one should ever be surprised that dearly held biologic constructs are often conventions requiring empiric confirmation.

21

An Epidemic of Hypercalcemia

"Once you eliminate the impossible, whatever remains, no matter how improbable, must be the truth."—Sherlock Holmes

MODERN MEDICINE IS RICHLY supported by a near infinite variety of laboratory tests. While running these tests may seem relatively harmless, the random performance of multiple laboratory tests on healthy individuals has a real possibility of generating a false positive signal of abnormality.

For example, if a panel of twenty tests are run on a healthy person, with each test designed to correctly identify a normal patient as normal 95 percent of the time, it can be expected that 64 percent of the time at least one of these tests will give a false indication of abnormality.

$$1 - .95^{20} = 64\%$$

It is for this reason that doctors should be judicious, ordering tests in a meaningful clinical context and only when needed. The whole point of a clinical examination and history is to establish clinical context, produce a reasonable differential diagnosis, and constrain testing to a limited subset of tests to minimize false positives.

When an unexpected result is reported, doctors often repeat the test to make sure that they are not seeing a false positive.

Now to the story.

A group of physicians in a Montefiore clinic began seeing moderately elevated blood calcium levels. Blood calcium levels are often routinely ordered in a panel of twenty laboratory tests. At first, they did not really appreciate what was happening. These were mild elevations, so they merely repeated the test expecting the calcium to be normal upon retesting. To their surprise the calcium levels remained elevated. Subsequent evaluation included radiologic evaluations and referrals to endocrinology.

Since individual physicians were not ordering a calcium test on every patient, each rarely experienced this "elevated calcium signal." The small number made it impossible for the individual physician to detect the "epidemic of high calcium" experienced by the clinic as a whole.

It was only the medical director of the clinic, looking at a pile of endocrinology consultation requests, who saw the big picture.

Now, calcium levels can be elevated by cancer, but none of the patients were found to have any cancer.

Calcium levels can also be elevated because of abnormal growth in the parathyroid glands—small glands in the neck that regulate calcium levels. But here, too, no abnormalities were found.

After repeated expensive workups, all failing to find pathology, the doctors turned to a possible, if unlikely, explanation. As Sherlock Holmes said, "Once you eliminate the impossible, whatever remains, no matter how improbable, must be the truth." Could it be that our superb reference lab was generating erroneous results? How could this be? The laboratory had impressive quality control and was constantly reviewed, evaluated, and certified by the laboratory accreditation program of the College of American Pathologists.

The medical director called the laboratory director, who reviewed the laboratory quality assurance procedures on the calcium instrument and found no abnormalities. He assured the medical director that all was in order.

The medical director, now chastened by the lab director's report confirming his own initial low expectation of a laboratory problem, returned to his daily duties and put the issue behind him.

Unfortunately, the next month, he once again found himself buried with endocrine consultation requests. Now his doctors were also aware of the situation and not happy at all.

Once again he reached out to the laboratory. Once again, a check of the laboratory quality assurance records revealed no abnormalities. Standard tests run on the laboratory calcium channel showed performance within tolerance, and an attempt was made to reassure him once again. This time, however, he was not reassured.

What should the medical director do?

Keep in mind that for the medical director, the possibility of a novel epidemic of hypercalcemia was not an "impossible" consideration. Montefiore in the early 1980s had experienced an "impossible situation" of an epidemic of wasting disease in young women. Unlike GRID (gay-related immunodeficiency disease), a similar disease appearing in the homosexual male community, this disease was appearing in heterosexual women. Ultimately, sexual transmission of HIV in drug users was identified as the common cause.[19] So this medical community, having experienced surprising epidemics in the past, did not ignore a potential outbreak pattern.

Fortunately, the medical director had access to Clinical Looking Glass. He could review all his clinic's patients over time, restricting analysis to the first calcium for each patient.

Question: Why is this a useful strategy?

Answer: By looking at how the number of "elevated first calcium" changed over time, the clinic director could make a thoughtful observation on the changing *incidence* of elevated calcium cases over time. He knew that his clinic had a reasonable number of elevated calcium cases six months and a year back. By looking at each patient's first elevated calcium result in these time periods, he developed an expectation of incidence of elevated calcium case rate to compare to his present experience.

His analysis showed a significant rise in the number of patients with elevated calcium in the present two months as compared to similar intervals six months and twelve months prior.

Armed with this new information, the medical director asked the laboratory for a more thorough test of the calcium channel. This look revealed that the chemistry machine for calcium had drifted and was inaccurately reporting hypercalcemia.

Why did the laboratory miss this problem before, and why did it detect the elevated calcium level now?

The clinicians had noticed that the hypercalcemia they were detecting was in the range of just above normal—10.5 mg/dl. However, as part of its quality assurance effort, the laboratory tested its calcium machines with controls whose values were at the extreme high and low range—not at the specific diagnostic decision cut point of 10.5. While the machine was performing well at the extremes, and it was at the extremes that the controls were evaluated, there was accuracy drift in the central region. In fact, the critical drift occurred in the very center of the diagnostic decision zone. It was only with specially requisitioned controls in the 10.5 to 11.0 range that the hidden drift was detected.

An astute clinician, building simple cohorts of patients in different time periods, unmasked a failing calcium channel, thereby ending an epidemic of anxiety and costly workup for a nonexistent epidemic.

22

BIG IS BETTER? BUT IS IT ENOUGH?

IN *THE EVERYTHING STORE: Jeff Bezos and the Age of Amazon*,[20] Brad Stone describes the way Amazon plows through customer purchasing history in response to changes in its advertising, manipulating fonts, style of messaging, and so-called adjacencies of products, all to change the number of goods sold. Amazon learns from these experiments and changes its marketing behavior from the knowledge gained to make phenomenal profits. This activity is called data mining and lives under the heading of Big Data.

Attached to the Big Data notion is a prevalent naïve notion of the "Wisdom of Crowds."[21] Crowdsourcing taps into the collective tastes and opinions of a large number of people. Even though individually no member of the crowd has any particular expertise, it is posited that by averaging the opinion of the uninformed, deep truths can be discerned. The concept eliminates the pesky need for education, the use of difficult statistics, or the experience gained by hard creative work of model testing and building a formal methodology. The advent of the Internet, with its ability to touch the opinions of millions at low cost, raised the expectation that if such a process could work, we could soon discover all.

While those engaged in the science of machine learning are actually quite a sophisticated bunch, taking advantage of any model or knowledge possible to enhance their capabilities, the ill-informed public imagination has embraced the notion of no pain–no brain–but big gain.

It has gotten to the point where some wealthy individuals[22] learned in a specific domain have suggested that all human knowledge and integrative ability will one day be replaced by a process that will open its colossal maw, ingest large volumes of raw data, and, *poof,* straw will be transmuted into gold. There is no limit to the claims made. Such a soothsayer is Vinod Khosla, cofounder of Sun Microsystems and now a venture capitalist betting on Big Data.

> "Sufficient data used properly and reduced to the right insights does in fact make up for errors. I would rather have 1,500 EKGs [electrocardiograms, a test that checks for problems with the electrical activity of the heart] done much more poorly than two EKGs done a year very well, because the sources of errors in the current system are just too large. When I have two EKGs a year, I may not be symptomatic. I'm not arguing that these systems don't have errors. I'm saying the volume of the data, properly applied, makes up for it."[22]

To be fair to Khosla, one should note the appropriate cautionary words: sufficient data, properly used, and properly applied. The problem, of course, is that the average reader does not see these caveats.

Incidentally, the choice of EKG is subtly biased to favor large number of measurements. The failure to extract information from an EKG is not merely due to the lack of human capability to properly interpret the test, but it is also due to the fact that the relevant finding might not have occurred to be detected in the short observation time of two EKG tests. The issue here is not quality of data extraction from an adequate sample. Two tests done over a total of thirty seconds is an inadequate sample of heart electrical activity for rare but important events when compared to hundreds or thousands of tests capturing seven thousand hours of electrical observation. It is this conflation of differing utilities of bigness without being explicit that adds to the public confusion—a public that would just as soon not be bothered by pesky details.

One of the great purported successes of crowdsourcing in medicine is the detection of epidemics of influenza. Historically, the Centers for Disease Control collected information in the form of viral culture results from certain sentinel virus laboratories. When the number of positive culture results went up, flu season was declared. This declaration remains important because it focuses public health efforts on vaccination and prophylactic treatment of suspicious case contacts in high-risk environments, such as densely housed elderly in nursing homes.

The idea of "Google Flu Trends" is fascinating. Is it possible to detect when the flu is entering into a community by scanning the searches by Google users for information about influenza and medications to treat symptoms? Could a surveillance system based upon social media usefully detect the presence of flu in advance of the culture results? Initial results were promising and generated extraordinary enthusiasm.

More recently, someone actually looked at the Google Flu predictions in the subsequent years, and found that they were abysmal. The Google Flu surveillance failure was ascribed to Big Data hubris.[23] Remember, hubris is human arrogance, which the Greeks believed their gods hated so much that they punished it with terrible consequences.

Part of the Google Flu failure is probably due to the changing Google proprietary algorithm, which is not stable year to year because it is constantly being optimized for Google's own business purpose, *not* for flu detection. Part of this may be due to the self-stimulation that occurs when the Google results are reported directly and indirectly to the public, generating a massive self-amplifying signal that does not exhaust.

Big Data has great promise, but it will require mature evaluation to obtain its promised benefits.

I also believe that at the end of the day, human knowledge is finite. Often you go to your doctor to get reassurance that what you are doing is reasonable. There is an element of the priesthood in the patient–doctor relationship, and until our knowledge becomes so complete that a machine can extract the information flawlessly from the patient, and then map it flawlessly to a single disease and perfect therapy, there will be a need for the social construct of doctor as priest-healer.

Population Health

The Socio-economic Status Trilogy

23

DOES LOW SOCIOECONOMIC STATUS PREDISPOSE TO HIGHER READMISSION RATES?

How Intervention Thwarts Attribution with No Good Deed Going Unpunished

SINCE REIMBURSEMENTS ARE SOON to be tied to performance (thirty-day readmission rates among them), many organizations with poverty-stricken patients fear that they will be penalized for social factors causal of readmission that are beyond their control. For example, a lack of home supports for daily living puts the poorer population at greater risk for readmission. A recent analysis at Detroit's Henry Ford Hospital[24] demonstrated a clear relationship between lower SES and an increased thirty-day readmission rate.

Question: In Montefiore in the Bronx, do we have evidence that poverty is associated with increased rates of readmission?

Answer: First, Montefiore needed a metric for socioeconomic status. Roux et al. provided such a metric based upon US census data for the census block in which a patient resides.[10] They built a measure that combines income, home value, education, occupation, and percentage of residents who have interest or dividend income in order to assign an SES score to each census block. We used this method to calculate SES scores for all New York State census blocks, determining for each census block its relative position to the state mean using standard deviation as the unit of measure. A greater number of standard deviations in the positive direction means richer. A greater number of standard deviations in the negative direction means poorer.

With this metric in hand, we attached a neighborhood SES indicator to each discharge and built statistical models evaluating SES on thirty-day readmissions. To refine our study, we built a cohort of patients with the following study criteria.

Cohort:

- inpatient discharges from Montefiore Medical Center, Bronx, New York
- discharged alive and not to hospice
- Medicare as source of payment
- age greater than or equal to sixty-five
- excluded diagnoses: lung, gastrointestinal tract, or unspecified cancer
- time:year 2010

Clinical Looking Glass documented our cohort-building rules automatically during the build; these rules can be found in Appendix 1 at the end of this chapter.

Outcome: Thirty-day readmission? (Yes/No)

Possible explanatory variables:

- socioeconomic status (definition found in Appendix 2 at the end of this chapter)
- age

- race (not White versus White)
- ethnicity (Hispanic versus not Hispanic)

Results:

In the year 2010, a total of 25,571 discharged patients met these criteria. Figure 4 shows the SES distribution.

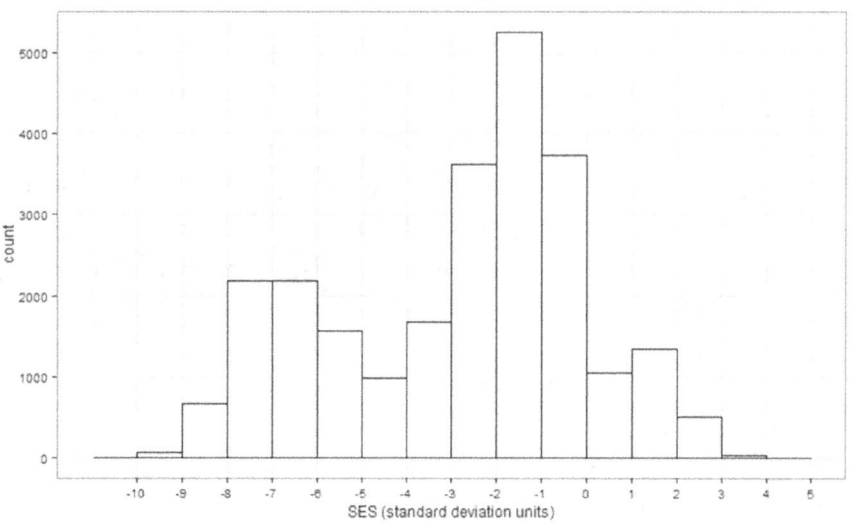

Figure 4. SES distribution of Montefiore Medical Center patients

Figure 4 is a histogram that shows the number of Montefiore patients with an SES index value between the two sides of the rectangle centered at the middle value. The New York State average SES is zero. You will observe that the bulk of Montefiore's patients are to the left of zero, so they are significantly poorer than the New York State average. The most frequent SES score is centered around –1.5 standard deviations below the New York State average.

Overall Thirty-Day Readmission

The next question to answer was what were Montefiore's readmission rates? Table 16 shows the cumulative percent readmitted by a specific day post discharge.

Table 16. Overall cumulative readmission rate by day at Montefiore Medical Center

	By day 3	By day 7	By day 10	By day 15	By day 25	By day 30
Cumulative readmission rate	5.1% (4.9, 5.4)	8.8% (8.5, 9.2)	11.1% (10.7, 11.5)	14.7% (14.3, 15.1)	20% (19.5, 20.5)	22.1% (21.6, 22.6)

By day fifteen, 14.7 percent of the discharged patients in 2010 were readmitted. By day thirty, 22.1 percent of the patients were readmitted.

We explored the impact of SES by reordering the discharges by their SES score from lowest to highest and dividing the list into five categories, or quintiles, with an equal number of discharges in each category.

Our resulting categories were:

- less than −6.17 (lowest level and baseline to which all were compared)
- [−6.17 to −2.73)
- [−2.73 to −1.3)
- [−1.3 to −.576)
- [−.576 to 3.88)

For non-specialist readers who are curious, the convention here is that the square bracket means "include the endpoint." A parenthesis means "do not include the endpoint."

Without going into too much statistical detail, we built relative risk models. These were statistical models that asked the question: Compared to the baseline of lowest SES status (less than −6.17, in our case), what was the relative risk of readmission as we moved to progressively higher SES statuses?

The models produced an estimate of the relative risk. If for higher SES levels the relative risk was less than one, then the higher SES was protective against readmission. If for higher SES scores the relative risk was greater than one, then the higher SES was associated with a higher readmission rate. In light of the findings at the Henry Ford Hospital, we expected to see rising SES scores associated with a progressively more protective effect—a relative risk of less than one at each level, and shrinking as we went up in SES value.

I provide the relative risk and 95 percent confidence interval for the relative risk model. A 95 percent confidence interval (from the 2.5th percentile to the 97.5th percentile) gives a sense of the variability of the relative risk estimate (Table 17). It is permitted to draw an inference on the readmission protective or exacerbating effect with rising SES only if the 95 percent interval excludes the value of one. A relative risk of one means that there is no difference in the readmission risk of the higher SES patients as compared to lower SES patients. By excluding one in the interval, the inferential statement of the relative risk is believable (i.e., less than one means protective, and greater than one means exacerbating, readmission rates).

In 2010 at Montefiore, males had a relative risk compared to females of 1.085 with a confidence interval (1.034, 1.139) excluding one, so we concluded that men were more likely to be readmitted than women (see table 17).

Table 17. Relative risk thirty-day readmission rate by SES in 2010 at Montefiore Medical Center

	Relative risk 30-day readmit	2.5%	97.5%
SES level			
SES < -6.17	Baseline	Baseline	Baseline
SES [-6.17 to -2.73)	0.976	0.902	1.057
SES [-2.73 to -1.3)	1.212	1.125	1.307
SES [-1.3 to -.576)	1.231	1.141	1.327
SES [-.576 to 3.88)	1.068	0.985	1.159
Gender:			
Female	Baseline	Baseline	Baseline
Male	1.085	1.034	1.139

The SES level <–6.17 is the baseline SES level against which all SES comparisons were made. SES for the next level up [–6.17 to –2.73) had a relative risk of 0.976. Since it is less than one, we saw a "protective effect," as we had anticipated. Rising SES reduced the readmission rate.

However, when we looked at the 95 percent confidence interval (from 0.902 to 1.057), we realized that the value one was included therein, so we were not permitted to draw any inference, as this observation was not statistically significant.

Going up to the next SES level of [–2.73 to –1.3), we were shocked to find a relative risk of 1.212. This relative risk is greater than one and suggested that higher SES was associated with more readmissions. The confidence interval of (1.125 to 1.307) excluded the value one, so the relative risk inference was believable and statistically significant.

The next level up [–1.3 to –.576) showed the same pattern of increasing readmission rates with higher SES—this finding was very surprising given the reported experience of Henry Ford Hospital, together with our naïve intuition that higher SES should be protective.

This is where we begin to develop longitudinal intuition. What might have been the cause of our inability to detect increasing readmission rates with lower SES?

There were at least five possibilities.

One, there simply may not have been a relationship between lower SES and increasing readmission rates. This defied our intuition and the Henry Ford Hospital study. But even worse, our data showed the reverse relationship. Why should people with better SES scores actually have increased readmission rates?

Two—mentioned only for the sake of completeness—is the possibility that our study had too few discharges so what we were seeing was the result of random chance. This is the classic statistical power argument: the sample size was too small to have a reasonable chance of detecting the effect we sought. Unfortunately, for this explanation, our sample size was huge (25,571), so we should have had sufficient power. Moreover, we *did* detect a statistically significant relationship. It just was in the wrong direction. Statistical power was not the issue.

By way of a third explanation, look at the SES distribution in Figure 4. You can see that most of the patients had SES scores below the mean of New York State. The mode (or most common value) was −1.5 standard deviations, and we had very few discharges on the positive side of two standard deviations. It might be that there was a relationship between low SES and readmission, but in order to benefit from rising SES, one must cross an SES threshold. Perhaps going from a horrendous SES to a merely horrible SES did not provide enough substantive advantage to remediate those socially determined causes of readmission.

So long as a patient was below this SES threshold, the protective effect of the higher SES level was not applicable. As the Henry Ford Hospital's SES scores, of course, were not standardized to the New York State norm, there was no way for us to judge whether the SES range at Henry Ford was broader than that of our model.

A fourth explanation recognizes that our hospital's information system did not reflect patient admissions to other hospitals in the Bronx. If lower SES patients tended to differentially seek other hospitals for their readmissions, those readmissions would be invisible to our analysis, making those patients seem to have fewer readmissions than the higher SES group. Was there some reason to suspect that this tendency was possible? Actually, yes. If one of the hallmarks of low SES is a chaotic, unpredictable day-to-day lifestyle, then perhaps that very disorganization extended to a patient's follow-up care, in which case the patient did not seek such care in any particular hospital for continuity, but rather sought it wherever he or she happened to be at the time.

Finally, a fifth explanation was very disquieting. The lower readmission rate might have been a subtle indicator of bad care for the poorest patients. Since only those who continue to live can be readmitted, if those with the lower SES had a higher mortality rate, then it was death that was preventing their readmission, not better care. Studying the death rate required that we account for all deaths, both within and outside the hospital. Fortunately in 2010, the Social Security Administration made its death tapes available to researchers, allowing us to know for all people with Social Security numbers whether they died in our hospital, in another hospital, or out of hospital.

Using this information as a resource, we found that in the first thirty days postdischarge, 4.2 percent of the patients died. Now we had to compare the death rates in different SES strata to determine if differential death rates could have accounted for the different readmission rates.

A rapid look at the mortality percentage by SES score rapidly disabused us of this concern (Table 18).

Lower SES did not have a higher death rate, so its lower readmission rate was not due to more deaths preventing readmission. In fact, surprisingly again, we saw *better* outcomes in the lower SES group. In building relative risk models comparing death rate to the lowest SES level, the three highest SES levels had statistically significantly worse death rates than the lowest one. Their relative risks were greater than one and the 95 percent confidence interval from 2.5 percent to 97.5 percent excluded one.

Table 18. Thirty-day death rate by SES status in 2010 at Montefiore Medical Center

SES level	30-day death rate
SES < -6.17	3.2%
SES [-6.17 to -2.73)	3.3%
SES [-2.73 to -1.3)	4.1%
SES [-1.3 to -.576)	5.1%
SES [-.576 to 3.88)	4.8%

As an aside, we saw that men were dying faster than women—1.4 times faster—which is a common finding (see Table 19). Women are the hardier sex.

Table 19. Relative risk thirty-day death rate at Montefiore Medical Center

	Relative Risk 30-Day Death Rate	2.5%	97.5%
SES Level			
SES < -6.17	Baseline	Baseline	Baseline
SES [-6.17 to -2.73)	1.00	0.81	1.24
SES [-2.73 to -1.3)	1.25	1.02	1.54
SES [-1.3 to -.576)	1.55	1.28	1.89
SES [-.576 to 3.88)	1.44	1.19	1.76
Gender			
Female	Baseline	Baseline	Baseline
Male	1.40	1.24	1.58

Could there be an encouraging explanation for why patients with the lowest SES seemed to be doing so well?

For the last fifteen years, our medical center has assumed a full-risk capitation approach focused on managed care and population health. Our care management organization uses a predictive model at discharge to identify the patients at highest risk for readmission, targeting them for follow-up calls and intensive care management. Therefore, if we have been successful both at identifying the high-risk patients and providing a meaningful intervention—and if low SES is correlated with high risk—our intervention efforts may have disproportionately targeted them. Our inability to show an SES relationship as intuitively expected may be a consequence of the success of our interventions. Hence, as in all research, looking for primary causes should be done before the intervention, not afterward. We have reason to suspect that our interventions are confounding the associations in a good way.

Appendix 1: Group Definition in Cohort-Builder Clinical Looking Glass

Group 1: discharges 2010 health affairs

Summary

Name: discharges 2010 health affairs
Description:
Number of Records: 25571
Type: EventCollection
Created On: 2014-05-13T20:33:00

Created By: ebellin6
Modified On: 2014-05-13T20:46:00
Modified By: ebellin6
Built On: 2014-05-13T20:46:00

INDEX EVENT : All Of Any

  Discharges [All Of *Discharges : InpatientDischargeDate* WHEN IN *2010* WITH *Age ge 65*]

Definitions list:
- Discharges : InpatientDischargeDate All

   Event Type: InpatientDischargeDate
   Not Disposition **InSet** 'USR:ExpiredOrHospice'
   And
   Line of Business **Equal** 'MEDICARE'
   And
   (...) Not InpatientICD9
       (
       Inpatient ICD9 Group InSet 'Cancer of bronchus; lung'
       And
       Position Equal 'Primary or Secondary'
)
   And
   (...) Not InpatientICD9
       (
       Inpatient ICD9 Group InSet 'Cancer of other GI organs; peritoneum'
       And
       Position Equal 'Primary or Secondary'
)
   And
   (...) Not InpatientICD9
       (
       Inpatient ICD9 Group InSet 'Cancer; other and unspecified primary'
       And
       Position Equal 'Primary or Secondary'
)

- 2010

   StartDate:01/01/2010 12:00 AM EndDate:01/01/2011 12:00 AM Start Date Included:true End Date Included:false

Figure 5. Group definition in Looking Glass

Appendix 2: Single-Created Variable to Represent Socioeconomic Status (for those mathematically inclined)

Source: Diez Roux, A.V., Merkin, S.S., Arnett, D., et al.: "Neighborhood of Residence and Incidence of Coronary Heart Disease." *N Engl J Med* 2001; 345(2):99-106.

The variables used in Montefiore's construction of a neighborhood socioeconomic score were selected on the basis of factor analyses of data from census-block groups. Factor analysis is a statistical technique that can be used to determine which variables out of a large set (for example, out of a large set of socioeconomic indicators obtained from the Bureau of the Census) can be meaningfully combined into a summary score.

Six variables representing dimension of wealth and income were combined into a summary score:
1. log of the median household income
2. log of the median value of housing units
3. percentage of households receiving interest, dividend, or net rental income
4. education (percentage of adults twenty-five years of age or older who completed high school)
5. education (percentage of adults twenty-five years of age or older who completed college)
6. occupation (percentage of employed persons sixteen years of age or older in executive, managerial, or professional specialty occupations)

For each variable, a z score for each block group was estimated by subtracting the overall mean (across all block groups in New York State) and then dividing by the standard deviation of all block groups in New York State. In our implementation, the z score reflects the deviation of the value from the mean of the population in New York State. For example, a score of 2.0 for the log of the median household income for a given block group means that the value for that block group is two standard deviations above the overall mean; a value of −2.0 is two standard deviations below the mean. The neighborhood summary score was constructed by summing the z scores for each of the six variables. For example, if z scores for the six variables for a given block group were 1.0, 1.5, 1.8, 2.0, 1.9, and 1.8, then the neighborhood score for that block group would be 10.0. Neighborhood scores for block groups in the sample ranged from −11.3 to 14.4, with an increasing score signifying an increasing neighborhood socioeconomic advantage.

The z score thus compares the SES of each individual against the New York State average.

For census data where the value was considered to be zero and a log of that value would have resulted in a negative infinity value, we substituted 0.5 for that value.

Take special note that a more careful analysis would assign to patients currently residing in nursing homes their last non–nursing home address. This study did not make a distinction between patients' nursing home addresses and their addresses of origin pre–nursing home.

24

I Am Too Poor to Benefit from SES Improvement

Threshold in the Service of Understanding

OUR PREVIOUS EFFORTS FAILED to find a relationship between rising SES and reduced readmissions. One potential explanation was that our patient population was, for the most part, too poor to show any impact. Could there be a threshold SES value that must be achieved before a rise in SES can manifest readmission rate reduction?

Using a validated census-based metric for neighborhood SES status,[10] the SES of all patients older than seventeen and discharged alive from an urgent or emergent Montefiore Medical Center admission from January 1, 2012, to April 30, 2014, were obtained with Clinical Looking Glass (see figure 6).

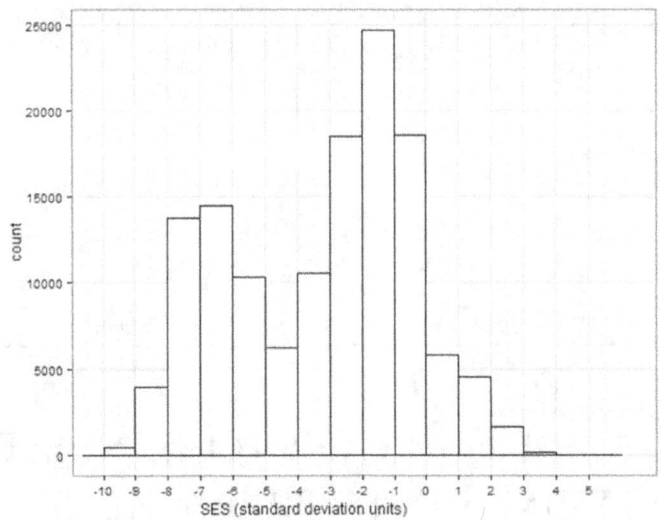

Figure 6. Histogram of SES by count, Montefiore Medical Center

SES values are in units of standard deviation from the New York State average, which is zero on the *x*-axis of figure 6. As you can see, the Montefiore population is skewed to the left, to the poorer population, with only 9 percent (12,044/133,666) above the New York State mean (SES = 0).

Recognizing that there might be a threshold before rising SES could be protective against readmission, we compared thirty-day readmission rates of patients whose neighborhood SES was greater than the New York State average to the readmission rate for those patients from SES neighborhoods below the New York State average:

- Thirty-day unadjusted readmission rate for Montefiore patients from neighborhoods with SES greater than the New York State mean was 16.9 percent.
- Thirty-day unadjusted readmission rate for Montefiore patients from neighborhoods with SES below or equal to the New York State mean was 18.2 percent.

We then built a risk regression model to adjust for other variables that might be responsible for the observed difference.

Controlling for age, dichotomized race (White baseline), dichotomized ethnicity (not Hispanic baseline), gender (female baseline), APR DRG weight (measure of intensity of care in the hospitalization as inferred from administrative diagnostic data using 3M Health Information System software), an SES greater than the New York State mean was protective against thirty-day readmission with a relative risk of only 90 percent of the lower SES group (95 percent confidence interval of 0.86, 0.94) (see table 20).

Table 20. Risk regression readmission model—dichotomous SES at Montefiore Medical Center

Variables	Relative risk	2.5th percentile	97.5th percentile
SES greater than New York State average	0.903	0.866	0.943
Age (linear)	1.002	1.002	1.003
Race (not White)	1.027	0.996	1.060
Ethnicity (Hispanic = yes)	0.991	0.968	1.102
Male versus Female	1.076	1.052	1.100
APR DRG weight	1.058	1.055	1.061

Patients with an SES greater than the New York State average were 10 percent less likely to be readmitted in thirty days than those below the New York State average.

Our previous inability to see the impact of SES might have been due to the fact that, as noted, most of our patients come from very low SES neighborhoods. The effect of increasing SES in a range of profound poverty cannot show an improvement in thirty-day readmission rates.

When the threshold value is crossed, in our case the New York State average, the 9 percent of patients from neighborhoods above this threshold demonstrate a statistically significant lower readmission rate than those below it.

25

INADEQUATE POWER OBSCURES FINDINGS

IN THE PREVIOUS SES studies, we used Clinical Looking Glass and the information in our electronic medical records to determine readmission rates. While the majority of readmissions return to our own institution, there is always the possibility that some patients will be admitted to other hospitals. Sole reliance upon our own information system would blind us to those admissions.

To study the impact of SES in a population in which all subsequent readmissions are known to us, we identified a population of discharges belonging to our managed care organization. These patients were all enrolled in a common managed care insurance program for which our care management organization was responsible for bill payment. Sensitivity to subsequent admissions to any hospital is therefore believed to be 100 percent. Hospitals tend to tell us about the admissions when it is the only way they are going to be paid. In this particular insurance product, in 2013, 6,006 patients had an admission. We evaluated the impact of SES on the risk for thirty-day readmission in these patients, adjusting for age, gender, and a proxy for "sickliness" based on diagnoses experienced in 2013.[25,26]

To start our analysis, we took advantage of our previous threshold analysis and dichotomized the admission population into two groups:

- 665 patients with SES greater than or equal to the New York State mean
- 5,341 patients with SES less than the New York State mean

We then performed relative risk regression modeling controlling for age, gender, line of insurance (Medicaid, Medicare, commercial), and a Clinical Risk Groups (CRG) weight (a measure of clinical severity based on administrative diagnoses). The results are summarized in table 21.

Table 21. Readmission relative risk regression at Montefiore Medical Center

Variables	Relative risk	2.5th percentile	97.5th percentile
SES greater than or equal to New York State mean versus SES lower than mean	0.733	0.594	0.905
Medicaid versus commercial insurance	1.305	1.085	1.568
Medicare versus commercial insurance	1.144	0.958	1.366
Age (linear)	1.009	1.005	1.013
CRG weight	1.032	1.029	1.035
Male versus female	1.073	0.966	1.193

SES above the New York State mean is protective against readmission with a relative risk of 0.733. This means that people coming from neighborhoods with an SES above the New York State mean are

27 percent less likely to be readmitted than those below the New York State mean. Patients receiving Medicaid (the medically indigent) are 1.3 times as likely to be readmitted compared to patients with commercial insurance.

Older patients are also more likely to be readmitted with Medicare patients 1.144 times, as likely as commercially insured patients to be readmitted. For every year of increasing age, there is a 0.9% increase in risk of readmission.

With increasing sickliness as manifested in diagnosis-based CRG weight, there is a higher likelihood of readmission. Note all these variables have a 95 percent confidence interval that excludes one with the inference that the findings are significant.

Gender has a confidence interval (0.966, 1.193) including one, so is not significant in contrast to the earlier model.

Another modeling strategy created matched sets of patients derived from the two SES groups. Each patient in the high SES group was matched with an appropriate patient in the low SES group, with patients reused if they were the best matches. Functionally it went like this. We took our first high SES patient and looked for its match in the low SES group. When we found a match within predefined tolerances (age within three years, same sex, CRG severity within 0.2), we put each of the pairs into their respective subgroup. We kept doing this, even reusing controls if there were not enough controls within the tolerances, until we could not find any more matches. The resulting two synthetic high and low SES groups constituted our best effort to create two subpopulations evenly balanced on all relevant variables (other than SES), so when we analyzed the impact of SES, all important confounders had been managed. Since all the potential confounders were balanced, the outcome difference between the two groups was attributable to SES.

The results are provided in table 22, with the characteristics in the two groups before and after the match, demonstrating excellent balance in the post-matched population.

Table 22. SES group characteristics before and after match

Variables	Before Match		After Match	
	SES ≥ 0	SES < 0	SES ≥ 0	SES < 0
Male	45%	39%	44%	44%
Average age	60	57	60	60
Severity of illness (CRG weight average)	4.6	5.0	4.0	4.0
Number of unique patients	665	5341	634	582

When we performed the matched risk regression analysis in the two synthetic populations using SES (high and low) as an explanatory variable, we found (to our horror) that SES was no longer significant.

At this point you must be ripping your hair out wondering when this analysis will ever come to definitive closure. However, this last example is critical to making the point that when you conduct a study, you need to know whether you have enough patients to detect a statistical difference, should one actually exist. As touched on earlier, this is the important notion of power.

There are equations to calculate power, but fortunately modern programs make this analysis trivial. One such statistical software program is "Power and Precision" (version 4) by Biostat.

To calculate power, you first need to estimate what effect size difference you are trying to detect.

If you look at the two groups of patients in our data set, you will find that the readmission rate of those with low SES was 0.180 (18 percent within thirty days). For the high-SES group, the readmission rate was 0.155 or (15.5 percent in thirty days). The effect rate difference was small at 2.5 percent.

How many people did we have to enroll in each arm of the study to have a power of 80 percent to find the observed difference of 2.5

percent with statistical significance -- to have an 80 percent chance of declaring the found reported difference significant?

Using the power program we determined that we needed 3,502 patients in each group (see figure 7).

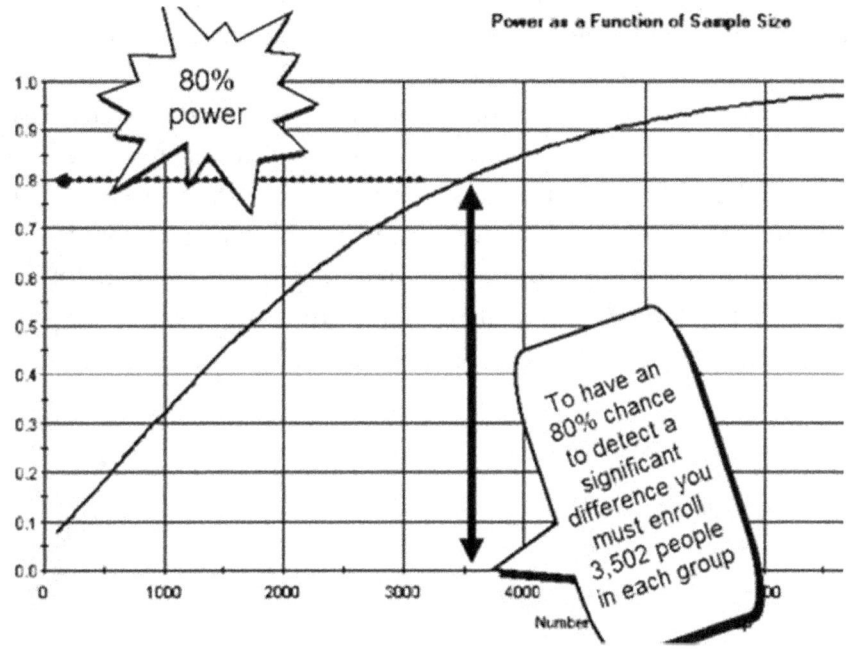

Figure 7. Power as a function of sample size.

After our matching process, we had only 1,216 patients total, not the 7,004 (3,502*2) patients required from our power calculations. This analytic strategy simply did not have adequate power to detect significance.

In summary, in a population of great poverty, when there was adequate sample size for risk modeling, we found that SES greater than the New York State mean resulted in fewer readmissions than in patients with an SES lower than the New York State mean. Power raised its ugly head when we reduced our sample size through our matching method below the numbers required to detect the effect.

Where do we go from here? Do we continue to analyze the SES to death? Some might say we already have. Or, having now recognized the vulnerability of this patient subgroup, do we begin to meaningfully problem-solve? Do we interview those patients from low SES upon readmission and try to tease out explicitly the remediable life challenges that can be anticipated at discharge? From a public policy perspective, this information can be used in one of two ways. The first use, from a report card perspective, could be to handicap hospitals serving poorer populations, forgiving them their poor readmission rates. The other use might be on an ongoing basis, to provide directed funding to survey their impoverished readmission population to discover the preventable, and then provide additional funds to address the problems discovered. It is important to know when to analyze, when there's been enough analysis, and when it is time to stop analysis and begin a focused intervention.

The Obesity Epidemic Trilogy

26

WHERE ALL THE CHILDREN ARE ABOVE AVERAGE

Lake Wobegon Meets Public Health

> "Where all the women are strong, all the men are good-looking, and all the children are above average."—Garrison Keillor

IN HIS RADIO SHOW, *A Prairie Home Companion,* Garrison Keillor creates a fictional town with a statistical paradox: "All the children are better than average."

We live in an incredibly self-affirming society. Everyone is excellent. No one is foolish. Every idea is valuable and worthy of consideration. Everyone is smart, handsome, strong, and beautiful. But even in our colossal narcissism, it is a logical impossibility for everyone to be above average.

Average has an actual, operational definition that cannot be wished away. To calculate an average, you must collect everyone's measure, add those values together, and divide that sum by the number of people. The result is the average. If the individual values are evenly distributed in the population, then we should expect that half the population should be above average and half below. Thus Lake Wobegon would not be able to sustain a population where the children are all better than average.

Question: How can we turn this joke into an instructive riddle? How *could* Lake Wobegon's children be better than average?

Answer: With a slight modification of phrase, we can eliminate the paradox. While Lake Wobegon's children cannot all be better than their own average, each child can be better than some other reference population's average.

The whole idea of a reference population is important when trying to make sense of health need priorities and need to contextualize the findings.

Let's consider a relevant public health question. We are in the middle of an obesity epidemic. More than 30 percent of the adult population in the United States is obese, which is a dramatic increase over the preceding decade. We want to intervene, and we want to intervene early, but who should be targeted? There is an obesity measure, BMI percentile, which takes into consideration height, weight, gender, and age. This measure is calculated for all children in a reference population, the BMI values are sorted from lowest to highest value, and the percentiles are determined by cutting the list of sorted values at the first 10 percent of the population (10th percentile), the first 20 percent of the population (20th percentile). A percentile is the value that is greater than or equal to the value seen in x percent of the population.

That means that the 60th percentile BMI is the BMI value greater than or equal to the BMI value seen in 60 percent of the reference population. The 95th percentile BMI is the BMI value greater than or equal to the BMI value seen in 95 percent of the subjects in the reference population. The top 5 percent of the population have a BMI value greater than or equal to this value.

Suppose you were evaluating a group of students in your child's school. You took all their BMIs, sorted the BMIs from lowest to highest, and then compared those BMI values to the percentiles in the reference population. If the population in the school had the same BMI value distribution as the reference population, you would expect that the 95th percentile value of your child's school would be the same as the 95th percentile value in the reference population. You would expect that the BMI value at the 75th percentile in this population would be greater than 75 percent of the BMI values in the reference population. However, if you found that the school population's 75th percentile value was the same as the reference population's 95th percentile value, you would have discovered that 25 percent of the children in your child's school have a BMI in excess of 95 percent of the children in the reference population. This would be a shocking and dramatic problem. This is also a problem that I actually observed.

Notice, I have not even told you whether in an absolute sense the children in the top 5 percent of the reference population are obese. But given that the reference population is the US population—and knowing that the United States is suffering from an obesity epidemic—you probably could safely conclude that if 25 percent of the children in your child's school have a BMI value greater than the United States' 95th percentile, the children in your child's school are quite fat.

The proper intervention and timing have yet to be determined. Should it be at age eleven, with significant increases in diet control and exercise targeting those already on their way to the ranks of the top percentiles? Should it be targeting those in their post–growth spurt? Should it be broadly applied? This is the challenge of our population's healthcare delivery system: to not only recognize the problem through comparison to the proper reference group, but also to target the appropriate group at the appropriate time in order to reduce the obesity epidemic. We do not want all our kids to be fatter than average.

27

Belching Fat

Fat Pollution—the Modern Scourge of High BMI

TO SOLVE A PROBLEM, you first have to develop a clear model of the problem. A clear image can help focus efforts, shape public policy, and mobilize interventions. When we think of the problem of air pollution, for instance, the image of a smokestack, belching dark smoke on helpless citizens, is a powerful visual aid to identify the risk and the potential target of intervention.

In modern society's battle of the bulge—a grossly overfed population now verging on 30 percent obesity nationwide—identifying the analogous "fat" smokestacks is critical.

Humans are genetically programmed to seek sweets and fat. These appetites have evolved over eons in calorie-poor environments among nomadic humans who eked out survival by gorging when calories were available and husbanding their resources when calories were not.

While our genes have not changed, the availability of calories has. We have built huge economic engines in agribusiness whose primary function is to capture more dollars from the sale of processed food products than from fresh foods. These businesses spend enormous sums testing ways to modify our behavior through advertisements, sponsorship of the activities we like, and creation of peer-group norms tapping into our natural gregariousness. The rapid processes of testing the social environment, measuring the sales impact, and then modifying the interventions are so ingrained in the marketing machine that as a society we are blind to its pervasiveness. Our public health and medical infrastructure is by comparison so seventeenth century.

The extent of the perfidy is obvious to any parent shopping at a supermarket. Marketing gurus put treats at the eye level of a child sitting in the child's seat of a shopping cart. Once seen, all hell breaks loose if Junior is not given his treat. And so begins the fattening of our population. This strategy continues as we get older, with companies competing for eye-level placement of their marketed calorie bombs on shelves.[27]

Where are the "fat" smokestacks in our world?

I propose the paradigm of thinking of the vending machine as a "fat-belching smokestack." It is hard to argue that the empty calories of candies, oil-soaked chips, hydrogenated fat-coated popcorn, and sugar-laced liquids in our well-fed society constitute anything other than fat pollution.

The innocuous vending machine in your office or school is a fat-belching polluter. It puts within easy reach empty calories and serves to enrich an industry intent on making money on the processing of raw food material. As that industry puts fat on our middles, our appetite for calories grows, and we enter a fat spiral from which few of us escape.

The first step to liberation is to identify the enemy and to identify the metric that must be used to monitor this insidious polluter.

I propose four metrics for each vending machine and for the collective of vending machines in any institution committed to healthcare or education:

- the number of calories (dumped per month into our ecosystem based on sales)
- the number of calories per item sold
- the number of those items sold
- the dollar yield from each machine

With these metrics, we can focus the public discussion and the private negotiations with the food industry.

If we could reduce the total number of calories belched into our environment, presumably there would be fewer male bellies hanging over their respective belts.

Ideally we would see the number of calories per item reduced so that even if the number of items sold stayed the same or slightly increased, the net result would be fewer calories.

Dollar yield per machine is an important metric in any negotiation with the food industry to reduce caloric pollution. If the food industry does not see a dollar loss, they can be "calorie agnostic." This is important from a coalition-building perspective. It is also important that we achieve fat pollution reduction from vending machines in a way that will not encourage people to seek other sources to augment their calories.

If institutions use these metrics and consciously pursue their reduction, we can hope that combined with self-imposed portion control, we can begin to tip the scales in our favor.

28

How Can We Be Getting Fatter when a Higher Percentage is Losing Weight?

WHEN STUDYING A SCHOOL health population of children younger than age fourteen, Montefiore came across an interesting paradox. Between school year 2012 and 2013, we noted that a higher percentage of overweight children reduced their weight to normal than the percentage of normal weight children who became overweight. Yet, overall, the overweight percentage of the population increased.

Question: How could both be true?

Answer: Careful review of the data revealed a clear explanation. We collected BMI values of children seen in school health clinics in two consecutive school years. We designated a child as overweight if he or she had a BMI greater than or equal to the 95th percentile of a national aged-matched group. If not designated overweight, the child was designated normal. Each child was assigned to one of four categories based upon the child's weight status in 2012 and weight status is 2013. The total number of children who were so categorized is provided in table 23.

Table 23. Weight status of a cohort of schoolchildren studied in two consecutive school years by Montefiore Medical Center

2012 weight status	2013 weight status	Number of children
Normal	Normal	1,720
Overweight	Normal	95
Normal	Overweight	160
Overweight	Overweight	533

Now let's calculate.

15 percent (95/(95+533)) of the overweight became normal weight, while 8.5 percent (160/(160+1720)) of the normal became overweight.

But surprisingly, 25 percent ((95+533)/2,508) of the students in 2012 were overweight while 27.6 percent ((160+533)/2,508) of those same students in 2013 were overweight. So although the percentage of students losing weight exceeded the percentage of students gaining weight, the net population demonstrated a weight increase.

Question: How could this be?

Answer: The answer lies in realizing that in 2012 there were a lot more normal weight than overweight kids:

1,880 (1,720 + 160) versus 628 (95 + 533)

There were nearly three times as many normal-weight children as overweight children in 2012. Although the rate of change from overweight to normal was almost two times the rate of change of normal to overweight, the fact that the normal population of children was three times the number of the overweight children resulted in a net gain of overweight kids.

A strategy to reduce obesity will have to further increase the percentage of those who lose weight and reduce the percentage of those who gain beyond what is occurring naturally.

Silencing Death – The Unsolved Riddle

29

WHEN THE DEAD ARE SILENCED, WHO SPEAKS FOR THE LIVING?

Blind to One Million US Dead—How Public Policy for Healthcare is Thwarted

STARTING MONTHLY IN 2002, clinical quality experts could obtain the Social Security numbers of all those who died in the United States. Doctors and healthcare institutions concerned with patient safety and healthcare outcomes could marry institutional electronic health record data with Social Security death information.

However, in November 2011 the Social Security Administration (SSA) stopped releasing the Social Security numbers of 50 percent of the dead, making invisible the death of one million Americans annually. SSA receives death reports from family members, funeral homes, hospitals, states, death-aware federal agencies, and financial institutions, and it makes this information available to all federal agencies with a need-to-know. But Social Security policy makers, overturning a decade of practice, determined that the record of dead available from state reporting belonged to the states and the federal government had no right to redistribute it.

What did this change actually do to a hospital committed to information-driven accountable care, such as Montefiore?

Montefiore Medical Center is the only New York State participant in the Centers for Medicare & Medicaid Services (CMS) Innovation Center Pioneer Accountable Care Organization model. Montefiore is committed to a vision of population-based healthcare, focused on community outcome and patient safety.

Using Clinical Looking Glass, we determined that in 2010 Montefiore Medical Center and its outpatient facilities touched 499,148 unique patients. In a borough with 1.4 million inhabitants, this means that we touched 36 percent of the Bronx population, either in our outpatient or inpatient facilities.

Montefiore is unusual in its ability to analyze a population-based cohort. But even with so large a footprint and a deep commitment to quality and longitudinal care responsibility, Montefiore requires information from outside its own information system to be truly accountable for care.

Patients seek care outside our walls, and patients die elsewhere as well.

Over the past decade, mortality of Montefiore-admitted patients declined significantly. Using Clinical Looking Glass, we created cohorts of patients age sixty-five years or older seen for the first time in our largest division (Moses) in 2000, 2005, and 2010, and we followed them for a year. Twenty-five percent were age eighty-three or older and 10 percent were eighty-nine or older. Demographics are provided in tables 24 and 25.

Table 24. Gender by number, percentage, and year at Montefiore Medical Center

Year	Male	Female
2000 (baseline)	3,120 (40%)	4,706 (60%)
2005	3,513 (39%)	5,577 (61%)
2010	3,892 (38%)	6,249 (62%)

Table 25. Age percentiles at Montefiore Medical Center

Age	10th Percentile	25th Percentile	50th Percentile	75th Percentile	90th Percentile
Year					
2000	67	71	77	84	89
2005	67	70	77	84	89
2010	67	70	76	83	89

Using our hospital information system as the sole source of death information, cumulative mortality information for each of the three-year periods is provided in table 26.

Table 26. Cumulative mortality (hospital-based information at Montefiore Medical Center)

Year	By day 30	By day 60	By day 90	By day 180	By day 365
2000	5.0% (4.5, 5.5)	6.4% (5.8, 6.9)	7.3% (6.7, 7.9)	9.0% (8.4, 9.7)	11.1% (10.4, 11.8)
2005	4.3% (3.8, 4.7)	5.3% (4.9, 5.8)	6.1% (5.6, 6.6)	7.3% (6.8, 7.9)	8.9% (8.3, 9.5)
2010	3.4% (3.1, 3.8)	4.3% (3.9, 4.7)	5.0% (4.6, 5.5)	6.3% (5.8, 6.8)	8.2% (7.7, 8.7)

We noted a dramatic reduction in death—a relative risk of death of 0.71 (95 percent confidence interval: 0.65, 0.79) comparing year 2010 to 2000. We take great pride in this improvement, attributing it to heavy investments in information technology, safety initiatives, and rapid-response intensive care unit (ICU)-without-walls initiatives, among others. The rapid-response ICU-without-walls initiative created a highly trained team of critical care specialists available for rapid consultation at the bedside of any patient suspected of clinical deterioration. By not requiring admission to the ICU to obtain access to this level of expertise, we functionally made ICU-level care available outside the walls of the ICU.

However, even an institution with as large a geographical footprint as ours cannot be sure that it has captured all the deaths. How many die outside our walls? What is the impact of our palliative-care initiatives to properly support patients in their choice to die with dignity at home or in the care of a hospice? The only way to properly capture this information is to have access to a timely, universal death registry, and the closest we came to that prior to November 2011 was the Social Security death tapes.

Let's reexamine the Montefiore experience of combining mortality information from both the SSA and Montefiore electronic medical records (see table 27).

Table 27. Cumulative mortality (based on both hospital and SSA information at Montefiore Medical Center)

Year	By day 30	By day 60	By day 90	By day 180	By day 365
2000	6.6% (6.0, 7.1)	9.5% (8.8, 9.1)	11.7% (11.0, 12.4)	16.2% (15.4, 17.0)	22% (22.1, 22.9)
2005	6.1% (5.6, 6.6)	9.0% (8.4, 9.6)	11.0% (10.3, 11.6)	15.1% (14.3, 15.8)	20.8% (19.9, 21.6)
2010	5.0% (4.6, 5.4)	7.3% (6.8, 7.8)	9.3% (8.7, 9.8)	12.9% (12.2, 13.5)	18.0% (17.2, 18.7)

We continued to see a dramatic reduction in the death rate. The relative risk of death in the year following discharge comparing 2010 to 2000 was 0.79 (0.74, 0.85) confirmed in table 27 by the reduction in cumulative percentage mortality. However, now notice the mortality at 365 days. When we only had the mortality information from the hospital information system, the 2010 annual cohort mortality (table 26) was 8.2 percent as compared to 18.0 percent known from both the hospital and Social Security data.

For our accountable care initiatives and our efforts to look at the impact of new medications and interventions on patient outcomes, the presence of comprehensive Social Security death data is critical.

We have acquired the new Social Security death tapes and compared the number of patients identified from the Montefiore universe who died in the old tapes in 2010 to those who died in the de-enriched new release. We found a dramatic 50 percent reduction in death sensitivity.

What is the absurd result of this new Social Security policy change? Each institution committed to accountable care must contact each state and relevant municipality to obtain permission to get the Social Security death information. Each individual state's vital statistics group must fund a team of people to review these requests and then fund staff to create the data and distribute it. As if this were not enough, each state and relevant municipality must determine whether it can afford to do this monthly, annually, or not at all. In these extremely stressed financial times, just as the United States is on the verge of accepting norms of accountable longitudinal care using technology to improve health, a financial barrier has been created for no good purpose.

I do not know how this can be reversed. Can it reversed by presidential edict? By administrative reinterpretation? By legislative action that mandates a change in Social Security legislation to explicitly encourage the distribution of the death information monthly to institutions committed to serving the public health and safety? Will the national leadership protect the public interest?

Why try to universally fund healthcare while denying those charged with the program the death data necessary to improve quality?

This is a riddle I cannot solve, so I leave it to the activism and goodwill of my readers to appeal to Congress to pass a law requiring the sharing of death data from the Social Security Administration with healthcare entities responsible for promoting quality improvement.

The dead once contributed to the living. Now they are eternally silenced. I can only hope that our leaders in Congress and in the executive branch will not join the dead in their slumber.

About

30

About Advanced Analytics

WHEN YOU TRY TO solve a healthcare riddle, the first order of business is to frame the question properly. Define your temporally enriched cohorts. Define your outcomes. Decide whether you are looking for elapsed time to first event, density of events per unit time, presence or absence of a qualified event, or time a person spent in a specific range of laboratory values. These tasks are wonderfully delivered in Clinical Looking Glass. In a matter of minutes, we can use our electronic medical record's clinical information to simulate studies that would otherwise take months of chart review. We can compare results to clinical studies, and ask and answer questions that have just occurred to us.

Sometimes, however, we are challenged by the fact that our studies are observational in nature. We have not assigned therapies randomly to a group of patients. To compare two groups collected observationally and claim that the difference in outcome is attributable to a specific variable of interest, you must make sure that the two groups are comparable at baseline. For example, if you are comparing two groups of patients, one using drug A and another using drug B, before you can say that drug A has a lower mortality rate than B, you need to, control for age. If people taking drug A are younger than those taking drug B, the death outcome may be confounded by age—that is, the outcome of lower death rate is due to younger age, not the drug choice.

Advanced analytics can adjust for differences at baseline by either statistical modeling or by selecting for analysis only those patients in the two groups who match on variables thought to be related to outcome. Advanced analytics can permit you to analyze multiple outcomes per patient rather than a single outcome. Instead of assessing difference in readmission rates between groups using the presence or absence of a single first admission within thirty days of discharge, you might wish a metric to base its readmission rate comparison using all hospitalizations over a year's time.

This brief discussion cannot begin to cover all the details, but it can alert you to the existence of an exciting world of inquiry. I am actively working to make this capability easily available to my students and colleagues who build cohorts.

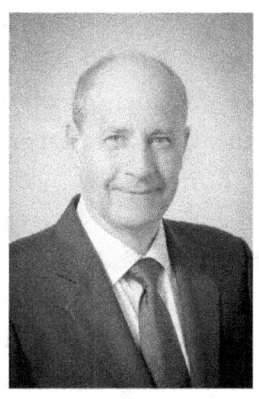

About Me

I GRADUATED FROM HARVARD College in 1978 with an A.B. in Chemistry and Physics. I attended medical school at Columbia University's College of Physicians and Surgeons, where I had the good fortune to meet Raymond Gambino, MD, in my second-year pathology course. Dr. Gambino had just published *Beyond Normality*[28] and introduced us to notions—then new to medicine—of sensitivity, specificity, and the impact of prevalence of disease on the meaning of a positive laboratory test finding. Dr. Gambino dramatically engaged his students in his senior pathology elective to generate hypotheses and test them. He had us look at the laboratory tests and predict what the patient would look like. He then had us look at the chart and ask how our impressions changed. We would then go to the bedside for the final intellectual reconciliation.

He brought us to MetPath, a major vendor of laboratory services to physicians, and showed us computer output of the distribution of GGTP lab test results for New York and northern New Jersey. GGTP is an enzyme released by an inflamed liver. He showed a year's worth of data and asked why there was a peak of elevated GGTP near the end of the year and beginning of the next? Any ideas?

The peak matched holiday cheer. Alcohol-soaked celebrations irritated the livers of the northern New Jersey crowd. This was my first experience with population laboratory test-based inference.

Amazingly creative and engaging, he was the quintessential teacher with a riddle. I was privileged to have known him.

After medical school, I served three years as a medical resident at New England Medical Center—an institution committed to longitudinal care. This was one of the last programs to allow each resident to follow his or her patient from the emergency room, to the hospital bed, to the intensive care unit, and back to the hospital floor. The notion of complete continuity was key. Follow-up continued into the outpatient experience, where the practice was shared in a one-to-one relationship with a nurse practitioner. Hospital service was organized by specialty. This was an incredibly collaborative place, where, for example, on the cardiology service, a doctor of pharmacology and nurses participated in daily work rounds with house staff to develop patient diagnostic and care plans. Maintaining a problem list was a near-religious requirement, with pride of place going to those residents whose problem lists made chart review a breeze. As residents, our intake notes and discharge notes were anchored by this highly curated clinical data summary.

Following medical residency, I took a Robert Wood Johnson Fellowship in Clinical Epidemiology at Yale under the direction of the formidable Alvan Feinstein, MD. He taught us research methods and design and luxuriated in creative neologisms. Dr. Feinstein coined a special phrase to describe a cohort of patients built from data retrospectively: trohoc.

For those who missed it, "trohoc" is the word cohort spelled backward.

He believed fiercely that a medical record, properly mined, could provide deep insights and serve as a real-world textbook of medicine. If he were alive today, I am sure he would see in Clinical Looking Glass echoes of his vision.

By the end of my epidemiology fellowship in 1987, the AIDS epidemic was in full force in New York City. Being a newly trained epidemiologist and witnessing the epidemic of the century, I could not sit this out. I sought and was accepted to a fellowship in Infectious Diseases at Montefiore Medical Center under Neal Steigbigel. The faculty, including Gerald Friedland and Robert Klein,[19] were among the first to describe heterosexual HIV transmission. As Montefiore ran the medical care program for inmates at Rikers Island jail in New York City, I had the opportunity to develop standards of AIDS and tuberculosis care—the twin epidemics of the late 1980s and early 1990s.

Upon completion of my fellowship, I worked at Rikers Island Health Service as the director of infectious disease services. At any one time there were 16,000 inmates cared for by 1,100 staff, inclusive of doctors, psychiatrists, psychologists, nurses, and mental health social workers. We built a 140-bed respiratory isolation facility for inmates with tuberculosis or suspected of active infection, and instituted a program of supervised TB therapy. Twice weekly patients were observed taking their medication, and at discharge they were connected with services in the community. Together with our partners in the department of health and other health organizations in New York City, we brought nine-month therapy completion rates to the mid-90 percent point. This was accomplished in a population previously unable to complete even four months of therapy with any reliability.

My colleagues and I built *The Bridge*: a computer application that tracked clinical data of inmates - a harbinger of our later work with Clinical Looking Glass.

In 1993 I became the program director of Montefiore Rikers Island Health Program. With a dedicated staff, including a creative and hardworking epidemiologist and analytically astute research analysts assigned to medicine, nursing, and psychiatry, the leadership and staff of the Rikers Island Health Service won Joint Commission on Accreditation of Healthcare Organizations accreditation with commendation—a first for a jail. It was during this tenure that I experienced the joys and challenges of running a clinical health delivery system. Subsequent analytics have been informed by my experience both as a doctor and chief executive officer of a healthcare delivery system responsible for longitudinal care.

In 1998 I returned to the Montefiore main campus. Montefiore had invested $50 million in an electronic medical record system covering both inpatient and outpatient facilities. Senior leadership, to their chagrin, discovered that while the electronic medical records they installed could provide detailed information on an individual basis, it was incapable of cross-patient temporally enriched analytics. This profound lack of capability continues to bedevil clinical information systems in current commercial use, and it encouraged Montefiore to support my efforts in building Clinical Looking Glass. I was fortunate that Montefiore had the vision to realize that the future of medical care was in capitated longitudinal population health responsibility, and that building a tool to support such a philosophy—as well as its triple mission of healthcare, research, and education—was critical.

Fifteen years of leading a programming team, teaching fellows and faculty, and internal consulting in epidemiology, quality, and healthcare administration has culminated in the realized Clinical Looking Glass program being deeply integrated into the triple missions and serving as a model for what analytics should look like in this space. Healthcare riddles are solvable with the right mind-set and tools.

Epilogue

About Montefiore Medical Center, Bronx, New York

HOW DO YOU SUMMARIZE an enormous socially committed organization in a few paragraphs? I provide a brief impressionistic overview of a remarkable institution with a remarkable history.

The Montefiore of the last twenty-five years, in which these tools and approaches gestated, was made of four hospitals with a total of 1,491 beds. In 2013 Montefiore provided 89,974 discharges, 320,886 emergency department triages, and 2,902,183 outpatient visits. Earlier in this book I introduced a metric of clinical activity known as "unique patients touched by Montefiore." As a reminder of that section, a patient is touched if he or she has experienced an emergency department triage, a hospital admission, an outpatient clinic visit, a laboratory test, or an outpatient prescription. In 2013, 492,993 unique patients were "touched by Montefiore" in a borough of 1.4 million.

Montefiore established a care management organization to take full-risk capitation, at present with 225,000 covered lives. Tightly affiliated with the Albert Einstein College of Medicine, and with one of the largest residency programs in the country, Montefiore is engaged in a triple mission of care delivery, education, and research.

Novel programs in school health, lead-poisoning prevention, and child-abuse prevention, with demonstrable outreach to the community, make Montefiore a real community player.

A remarkable group of socially committed practitioners and administrative leaders are continuously exploring ways to evaluate and improve care. The goals and needs of their patients have been the motivation for the analytics described in this book.

It has been and continues to be a privilege and honor to serve with them. I hope that this book will enable others to engage in clearer thinking as they assume longitudinal population healthcare stewardship.

BIBLIOGRAPHY

1. Roueché B. *Eleven Blue Men, and Other Narratives of Medical Detection.* Boston, MA: Little; 1953.
2. Levitt SD, Dubner SJ. *Freakonomics: A Rogue Economist Explores the Hidden Side of Everything.* New York, NY: William Morrow; 2005.
3. Gladwell M. *Outliers: The Story of Success.* New York, NY: Little, Brown and Co.; 2008.
4. Gladwell M. *The Tipping Point: How Little Things Can Make A Big Difference.* Boston, MA: Back Bay Books; 2002.
5. Houck PM, Bratzler DW, Nsa W, Ma A, Bartlett JG. Timing of antibiotic administration and outcomes for Medicare patients hospitalized with community-acquired pneumonia. *Arch Intern Med.* 2004; 164(6): 637-644.
6. Wachter RM, Flanders SA, Fee C, Pronovost PJ. Public reporting of antibiotic timing in patients with pneumonia: Lessons from a flawed performance measure. *Ann Intern Med.* 2008; 149(1): 29-32.
7. Deshmukh VG, Meystre SM, Mitchell JA. Evaluating the informatics for integrating biology and the bedside system for clinical research. *BMC Med Res Methodol.* 2009; 9:70.
8. Bellin E, Fletcher DD, Geberer N, Islam S, Srivastava N. Democratizing information creation from health care data for quality improvement, research, and education: The Montefiore Medical Center experience. *Acad Med.* 2010; 85(8): 1362-1368.
9. Mostel Z, Karnilova M, Arthur B, et al. *Fiddler on the Roof.* 1964.
10. Diez Roux AV, Merkin SS, Arnett D, et al. Neighborhood of residence and incidence of coronary heart disease. *N Engl J Med.* 2001; 345(2): 99-106.
11. Caro RA. *The Power Broker: Robert Moses and The Fall of New York.* New York, NY: Vintage Books; 1975.
12. Jencks SF, Williams MV, Coleman EA. Rehospitalizations among

patients in the Medicare fee-for-service program. *N Engl J Med.* 2009; 360(14): 1418-1428.
13. Weinberger M, Oddone EZ, Henderson WG. Does increased access to primary care reduce hospital readmissions? Veterans Affairs cooperative study group on primary care and hospital readmission. *N Engl J Med.* 1996; 334(22): 1441-1447.
14. Shear MD, Joachim D.S. V.A.. Chief Eric Shinseki, set to meet Obama, apologizes for "systemic" crisis. *New York Times.* May 30, 2014.
15. Shear MD, Oppel RA, Jr. V.A. Chief resigns in face of furor on delayed care. *New York Times.* May 30, 2014.
16. Hoover DR, Crystal S, Kumar R, Sambamoorthi U, Cantor JC. Medical expenditures during the last year of life: findings from the 1992-1996 Medicare current beneficiary survey. *Health serv res.* 2002; 37(6): 1625-1642.
17. Clopper C, Pearson ES. The use of confidence intervals or fiducial limits illustrated in the case of the binomial. *Biometrika.* 1934; 26: 404-413.
18. Preliminary report: Effect of encainide and flecainide on mortality in a randomized trial of arrhythmia suppression after myocardial infarction. The Cardiac Arrhythmia Suppression Trial (CAST) Investigators. *N Engl J Med.* 1989; 321(6): 406-412.
19. Harris C, Small CB, Klein RS, et al. Immunodeficiency in female sexual partners of men with the acquired immunodeficiency syndrome. *N Engl J Med.* 1983; 308(20): 1181-1184.
20. Stone B. *The everything store: Jeff Bezos and the age of Amazon.* New York, NY: Little, Brown and Company; 2013.
21. Surowiecki J. *The wisdom of crowds: Why the many are smarter than the few and how collective wisdom shapes business, economies, societies, and nations.* New York, NY: Doubleday; 2004.
22. Lee SM. Vinod Khosla: Doctors cannot compete with machines. *San Francisco Chronicle: SF Gate.* May 23, 2014. http://blog.sfgate.com/techchron/2014/05/23/vinod-khosla-doctors-cannot-compete-with-machines/. Accessed June 29, 2014.
23. Lazer D, Kennedy R, King G, Vespignani A. Big data: The parable of Google Flu: Traps in big data analysis. *Science.* 2014; 343(6176): 1203-1205.
24. Hu J, Gonsahn MD, Nerenz DR. Socioeconomic status and readmissions: Evidence from an urban teaching hospital. *Health Aff.* 2014; 33(5): 778-785.

25. Quan H, Li B, Couris CM, et al. Updating and validating the Charlson comorbidity index and score for risk adjustment in hospital discharge abstracts using data from 6 countries. *Am J Epidemiol.* 2011; 173(6): 676-682.
26. Quan H, Sundararajan V, Halfon P, et al. Coding algorithms for defining comorbidities in ICD-9-CM and ICD-10 administrative data. *Med Care.* 2005; 43(11): 1130-1139.
27. Thaler RH, Sunstein CR. *Nudge: Improving decisions about health, wealth, and happiness.* Rev. and expanded ed. New York, NY: Penguin Books; 2009.
28. Galen RS, Gambino SR. *Beyond normality: The predictive value and efficiency of medical diagnoses.* New York, NY: Wiley; 1975.

www.ingramcontent.com/pod-product-compliance
Lightning Source LLC
Chambersburg PA
CBHW072009200526
45167CB00021B/452